S. Hrg. 113–638

THE CHILDREN'S HEALTH INSURANCE PROGRAM: PROTECTING AMERICA'S CHILDREN AND FAMILIES

HEARING

BEFORE THE

SUBCOMMITTEE ON HEALTH CARE

OF THE

COMMITTEE ON FINANCE
UNITED STATES SENATE

ONE HUNDRED THIRTEENTH CONGRESS

SECOND SESSION

SEPTEMBER 16, 2014

Printed for the use of the Committee on Finance

U.S. GOVERNMENT PUBLISHING OFFICE

94–479—PDF   WASHINGTON : 2015

CONTENTS

OPENING STATEMENTS

WITNESSES

ALPHABETICAL LISTING AND APPENDIX MATERIAL

IV

COMMUNICATIONS

THE CHILDREN'S HEALTH INSURANCE PROGRAM: PROTECTING AMERICA'S CHILDREN AND FAMILIES

TUESDAY, SEPTEMBER 16, 2014

U.S. SENATE,
SUBCOMMITTEE ON HEALTH CARE,
COMMITTEE ON FINANCE,
Washington, DC.

The hearing was convened, pursuant to notice, at 2:54 p.m., in room SD–215, Dirksen Senate Office Building, Hon. John D. Rockefeller IV (chairman of the subcommittee) presiding.

Present: Senators Wyden, Schumer, Stabenow, Menendez, Brown, Bennet, Casey, Enzi, and Portman.

Also present: Democratic Staff: Anne Dwyer, Professional Staff; Elizabeth Jurinka, Chief Health Advisor; and Jocelyn Moore, Deputy Staff Director. Republican Staff: Becky Shipp, Health Policy Advisor.

OPENING STATEMENT OF HON. JOHN D. ROCKEFELLER IV, A U.S. SENATOR FROM WEST VIRGINIA, CHAIRMAN, SUBCOMMITTEE ON HEALTH CARE, COMMITTEE ON FINANCE

Senator ROCKEFELLER. Good afternoon. My apologies for being late. There was a long discussion at caucus, several votes, and the discussions were important, actually. I will make my opening statement. I am very grateful to Senator Enzi for being here. He cannot stay a long time, but he is here, and that counts.

I have been on this Finance Committee for a long time, and I have chaired this subcommittee for a very long time. I really do not remember ever having had a meeting of it before. The previous chairman had a different philosophy than the present chairman, who likes his subcommittees to be active. This, I have to say without sentiment, will be the last Health Subcommittee hearing that I chair. The first and the last. I think that has a certain panache. [Laughter.] I could not think of anything more important than doing it on the Children's Health Insurance Program.

The year 2014 marks the 17th anniversary of one of the most successful programs for improving children's health care in the United States, which is the CHIP program. It is a marvel. Eight million American children and families look to CHIP for comprehensive and affordable health care coverage, including 40,000 children from my own State in West Virginia. I am not sure about Wyoming and Ohio. Wyoming would have lower numbers. Ohio would have higher numbers.

CHIP's success has played an essential role in cutting the number of uninsured children in half over the last 14 years, from about 14 percent to about 7 percent. That was as of 2 years ago. This kind of progress is something we should celebrate. We must continue to invest in CHIP so that we can celebrate many more of the program's milestones.

In 1997, Senators Kennedy and Hatch and I spent countless hours discussing how we could increase health care access for children in a way that members of both political parties could support, not only to pass the program, but to sustain it, to keep it going, which is what we are trying to do now. Creating this program has been one of the most meaningful things I have done in my career in public service. I just flat out say that. If you are helping 8 million children all across the country, how can that not be important? How can that not be important?

So, without congressional action, I say again, CHIP will run out of funding next fall, placing at risk the well-being of hundreds of thousands of children and pregnant women. I hope that the members of this subcommittee will not let that happen.

It is an interesting program, because the Governors, both Democratic and Republican, tend to like it because there is a lot of flexibility in the way they can allocate funds and work with the way it is carried out. So I do not think there are a lot of Republican Governors who are against it. I do not think there are many Democratic Governors who are against it. In this case, since so much rests with the States, I think that is important for our decision-making.

But, it will run out of funding next fall. CHIP is a game changer for millions of children. No other form of coverage provides the same level of specific and comprehensive pediatric networks at an affordable cost for working families.

The challenges that many children face are too similar to the ones I first saw when I was a VISTA volunteer in Emmons, WV, nearly 150 years ago. [Laughter.] Every sight I saw there, Chairman Wyden, has stayed with me—every sight I saw there. Like when we went to Sago. I remember the look in your eyes as you listened to those families. Experiences like that make for lifetime commitments.

When I first arrived as a VISTA volunteer in Emmons, there were children in the town and across the State who had never seen a doctor because their families simply did not have the money to cover the cost of a physician visit or dental care. Dental care was out of the question. The wonderful thing about CHIP, generally speaking, is its coverage is better than that in the Affordable Care Act, which I do not like to say, but I have to in order to be honest. I thought then to myself, as I still do now, that no parent should have to carry the stresses of knowing that you cannot afford care for your children if something goes terribly wrong, and something goes terribly wrong very often with children in these rural areas and poor areas, which my State basically is.

I am proud to say that ever since CHIP's inception, the program has consistently enjoyed strong bipartisan support. One member of the Finance Committee, Senator Hatch, has remained a steadfast champion of CHIP from the very beginning. We have shared a goal of making certain that every child in America gets a fair shot at a healthy start in life. While we have not always agreed on every provision in the CHIP program, I have always appreciated Senator Hatch's strong, fundamental commitment to it.

For as long as I can recall, Congress has been able to, Mr. Chairman——

Senator WYDEN. You are Mr. Chairman.

Senator ROCKEFELLER. I am glad you are here, very glad.

Congress has been able to put aside its differences and come together when it was called upon to do what is right for American children. That time has come again, otherwise we will run out of money, and we will put the States into total disruption if they are not able to plan. You are going to help us understand that.

CHIP is currently at a crossroads. Funding for CHIP must be reauthorized soon, otherwise the program as we know it will come to an end, and as many as 2 million children could lose their coverage. This would threaten their health and their well-being, not to mention the significant gains that we have made over the past 17 years to reduce the number of uninsured children in this country. We simply cannot afford to take this major step backwards and jeopardize the future of generations by allowing CHIP to expire. We cannot do it. We just cannot do it.

If it was a matter of high controversy, that would be one thing—Republicans and Democrats clawing at each other's eyeballs, et cetera—but that is not the case. It just is not the case on this one. We do coalesce around children. This is a good bill. It has helped. It has done even what the Affordable Care Act has not been able to do.

A recent study by Wakely Consulting Group demonstrated that moving children into other forms of private insurance would cause a tenfold increase in out-of-pocket spending for CHIP families who cannot afford that. We just cannot have that. It is not right to shift the added financial burdens onto working families when a cost-effective solution for maintaining the coverage they already have exists.

Although funding for CHIP expires in 2015, the program is authorized through 2019. Now that is one of those anomalies that we produce sometimes in Congress. It usually helps, but if it does not, it is really bad. In other words, it is wonderful if the program is authorized, but it does not mean much if the money is not there. So, although the funding for CHIP expires in 2015, the program is authorized through 2019, which therefore could lead to significant disruption to State governments, private health plans, hospitals, and numerous other stakeholders, in addition to the families whose children are enrolled in the program. States have been budgeting and planning under the assumption that Congress would extend funding for another 4 years. They simply are not prepared to rapidly develop and implement plans to transition millions of children into other forms of coverage. In short, State legislatures and budget officials are relying on us to act now.

Colleagues, let us do our job. Let us show the American people that we can work together, that we can do something good. With that, I lay my case on the mercy of the subcommittee, the full committee, and the Congress.

[The prepared statement of Senator Rockefeller appears in the appendix.]

Senator ROCKEFELLER. Senator Enzi?

OPENING STATEMENT OF HON. MICHAEL B. ENZI, A U.S. SENATOR FROM WYOMING

Senator ENZI. Thank you, Mr. Chairman. I want to thank you for holding this hearing on a very important issue in health care. We may not always agree on every health care bill that comes before us, but we certainly can agree that the health of our young people is vitally important to our health as a Nation. You have made children's health the cornerstone of your career in the Senate, and I applaud you for your effort in raising the profile of this issue. I hope that your last hearing is your most productive hearing. [Laughter.]

I want to reiterate again, you mentioned that the Children's Health Insurance Program, CHIP, has been extended through 2019, but the funding only through September 30, 2015. So this hearing is intended to focus on the fact that the program funding will expire and needs extension.

We will draw attention to the administrative burden on States and the logistics and planning that require action sooner rather than later. I am pleased that we have such a distinguished panel to do that. The CHIP program is a valuable option for children who need health insurance, and I would like us to focus more on the core mission of the program in a way that builds on the good that many States are doing and which serves the population that truly needs help.

Wyoming's Kid Care CHIP is an example of targeting kids who are really in need and building a program that leverages the best of the public and private sectors to get children who do not have any other options the coverage that they need. That program is doing well, partly because of the flexibility that is allowed under this.

In 2003, Wyoming formed a public/private partnership with Blue Cross Blue Shield of Wyoming and Delta Dental of Wyoming to provide the health, vision, and dental benefits in Wyoming. All children enrolled in the program will receive a wide range of benefits including inpatient and outpatient hospital services, lab and x-ray services, prescription drugs, mental health and substance abuse services, durable medical equipment, physical therapy, den- tal, and vision services. The families do share in the cost of their children's health by paying copayments for a portion of the care that is provided.

I am hopeful that we can have a very positive dialogue about the path forward for CHIP. I think one of the greatest things that this program has is the flexibility. I hope that we continue that. We need to focus our efforts here on identifying the core mission of the program in a way that builds on the good work that many States are doing and what serves this population that truly needs help.

I appreciate the testimony of the people who are here. I have read through that and am impressed, and I hope that you will allow us to submit some questions when we cannot be here so that we can get additional information to get this right. So again, I thank you for holding this hearing.

Senator ROCKEFELLER. I thank you, sir.

[The prepared statement of Senator Enzi appears in the appendix.]

Senator ROCKEFELLER. The chairman of the full committee, Senator Wyden.

OPENING STATEMENT OF HON. RON WYDEN, A U.S. SENATOR FROM OREGON, CHAIRMAN, COMMITTEE ON FINANCE

Senator WYDEN. Chairman Rockefeller, thank you very much for doing this. I want to commend you and Senator Enzi for bringing us together to talk about this important program. Colleagues, I think it is worth noting that, at a time of extraordinary dysfunction and polarization here in Washington, this is a program where there is a consensus that it genuinely helps people in need, and particularly our vulnerable children.

This is medical care. It is dental care to millions of kids nationwide who otherwise, without CHIP, would be falling between the cracks. In particular, it has reduced disparities in health coverage for economically vulnerable Americans.

I just want to take a couple of minutes to note how we have arrived at this point, because you do not see a consensus built for an incredibly important program for vulnerable people by osmosis. It just does not happen that way. This program has come together because of the extraordinary leadership of Chairman Rockefeller. We certainly had Senator Hatch all of these years, and he was in your corner, Chairman Rockefeller, but make no mistake about it: this has come about because a humble person who has been relentless, relentless in his admirable desire to stand up for those in need, said he was going to go to bat for this program every step of the way, and that is why this program is on the books, Chairman Rockefeller. This is a particularly meaningful day, and we are going to have other times, colleagues, to talk about the great contributions of Chairman Rockefeller, what he has done to protect the retirement security for miners. I sat next to him, have for years, in the Intelligence Committee. None of you can know that because that is kind of classified. [Laughter.]

He did extraordinary work on cyber-security back when I had a full head of hair and rugged good looks and was director of the Gray Panthers. We passed petitions, actually, for work that Chairman Rockefeller did for seniors in terms of home health care.

We take a few minutes today to recognize what he has done for those who are vulnerable, and that legacy is going to continue. That legacy is going to continue in the days and years ahead, that legacy of grace, tenacity, and particularly making sure that, every time debates are conducted here in the Finance Committee and in Washington, DC, those without power, those without clout, those without political action committees, have a big voice. That is what Chairman Rockefeller's legacy is all about, standing up for those people.

I am going to have a chance to talk about other aspects of his career. I am particularly pleased that he is the leader of the Tall Senator's Caucus. [Laughter.] That is kind of meaningful to me, and I want to note one other point before I wrap up, and that is Chairman Rockefeller's selfless decision to decline the opportunity to chair the full Finance Committee, which allowed me to accept this position and the responsibility that goes with it. We all understand that Chairman Rockefeller would have been a superb chairman of the Finance Committee. I just want you and colleagues here to know that my gratitude for that selfless act, Chairman Rockefeller, is profound.

My goal here in the Senate Finance Committee is going to be to try to live up to the standards that you have set during your time in public service. Thank you.

Senator ROCKEFELLER. That is pretty nice. [Laughter.]

Actually, I was really happy as the chairman of the Commerce Committee. I am really happy that you are here.

Senator Brown?

OPENING STATEMENT OF HON. SHERROD BROWN,
A U.S. SENATOR FROM OHIO

Senator BROWN. Thank you, Mr. Chairman. I appreciate the chance to say a couple of words, first about you and second about this issue which is so very important. I do not speak for others, but I know that others agree with this, that Senator Rockefeller has been a friend and a mentor to me. He has taught me a great deal about translating human need into action in what this committee has done.

I am a relatively new member of this committee. I have been on—as has Senator Casey—for less than 2 years. I welcome the chance to help in a leadership role to build on the legacy of Medicaid and on CHIP that Senator Rockefeller has established in more than 2 decades on this committee. The work he has done, I followed that when I was in the House, saw what he did, and then got to work up close with him.

My State's CHIP program, fortunately for us I guess, is an extension of Medicaid. Kids will continue to receive coverage if funding is not authorized. We also know, though, that that means significant budget cuts. The type of cut is more cost-shifting to the States.

One thing I think we have learned is, we cannot keep doing that with Medicaid. We have also learned that Medicaid payment equity expires at the end of the year. We have made some progress in leveling the field between Medicaid and Medicare payment. That is something we need to continue. I think there is bipartisan support, too, for that.

Most importantly, Senator Rockefeller, thanks for making a difference in the lives of a lot of children on the other side of the Ohio River, on the north side, in addition to the south side of the Ohio River. Thank you.

Senator ROCKEFELLER. Thank you, Senator Brown. My only regret is that West Virginia owns the Ohio River. [Laughter.]

Senator BROWN. Which is actually true.

Senator ROCKEFELLER. Yes. I built eight bridges across, but you guys just put up about 20 cents.

Senator BROWN. Right.

Senator ROCKEFELLER. We had to carry the whole load.

Senator BROWN. I just think if you have a Rockefeller and a Brown, that Rockefeller puts up 80, Brown puts up 20. [Laughter.]

Senator SCHUMER. Let us have no class warfare here, Sherrod.

Senator ROCKEFELLER. That is right. Logic rules.

Okay. Senator Casey?

OPENING STATEMENT OF HON. ROBERT P. CASEY, JR., A U.S. SENATOR FROM PENNSYLVANIA

Senator CASEY. Mr. Chairman, thank you very much. I would want to incorporate by reference much of what Chairman Wyden said, as well as Senator Brown, in their praise of your public service and also your work for children.

There is an old expression about being summoned to give testimony at some point in our lives, and whenever Jay Rockefeller has been summoned to give testimony, it was almost in every case about kids, fighting and fighting and fighting on their behalf and, as Senator Brown mentioned, the Children's Health Insurance Program as well as Medicaid, two vitally important programs.

The chairman served as Governor. I want to mention another Governor, my father. After losing three times for that office, on his fourth try he won, and Pennsylvania was one of the first States to enact a Children's Health Insurance Program that became the national model, which you led with your colleagues.

I think, Mr. Chairman, we will have longer statements for the record about the benefits of CHIP. Let me just read you this, then I will conclude. This is from one of the families giving their own testimony about CHIP. ''The CHIP Program has been great. We know that there is quality insurance, and we are finally able to sleep at night knowing that our kids can be seen by excellent pediatricians. I do not know what we would have done without CHIP. Now my children can play sports and go away to camp like other kids, and, if they get hurt, CHIP is there for them.''

I could not, if I had an hour, say it better than that. That testimony is evidence of the benefit of the program, but also I think it is proof positive of your achievements in public service, especially for our kids.

Thank you very much.

Senator ROCKEFELLER. Thank you, Senator Casey. Senator Portman was here, and I am glad he was, because he is for this.

And now, Senator Schumer, if you can overcome your shyness, sir, you are on.

OPENING STATEMENT OF HON. CHARLES E. SCHUMER, A U.S. SENATOR FROM NEW YORK

Senator SCHUMER. Unaccustomed as I am to public speaking—— [Laughter.]

We could use a lot of nice adjectives for our dear friend Jay, whom we are so sorely going to miss. But let me just read you one sentence that would be greater testimony to him from my State of New York than all of the adjectives in the world.

When CHIP was enacted, New York had over 800,000 uninsured children. Today that number has decreased by 90 percent—what a legacy—all because of one person, Jay Rockefeller. His passion, his strength, and his caring have just been amazing. They have been an inspiration, I think, to many of us here in the Senate. Whether we had to fight the fights on the health care bill or in the CHIP program or throughout the appropriations process, there was no voice that was stronger or more effective than Jay Rockefeller's on behalf of kids and all of the voiceless in this country.

Just on a more serious note, as Sherrod was saying, that somebody who came from a background of plenty could care so much for the people who had nothing and then accomplish so much, is still a testament to the greatness of America. So anyone who doubts the future of this country, look at the biography and accomplishments of Jay Rockefeller, and you will feel really good about the United States of America and about him. Thank you.

Senator ROCKEFELLER. I am getting confused here. I am not going to break out into tears because I do not do that, but I really thought this was a hearing about CHIP. [Laughter.]

Senator SCHUMER. CHIP equals Rockefeller.

Senator ROCKEFELLER. All right. If I am going to hand out chances for punishment, I should certainly recognize Senator Menendez.

OPENING STATEMENT OF HON. ROBERT MENENDEZ, A U.S. SENATOR FROM NEW JERSEY

Senator MENENDEZ. Well, thank you, Mr. Chairman. I am going to be brief, but I hope that in your modesty you will not continue to use humor to deflect the praise that is coming your way.

I think that if I would sum up the lifetime of work that you have led here in the Senate, it is as a champion of children—children in the CHIP program, children in poverty, children in foster care. The people and the children of West Virginia, and for that matter, the children of the Nation including my home State of New Jersey, are better off because of Jay Rockefeller and his mission in life to help, as Senator Schumer said, the most vulnerable.

Nearly a generation now of children have received the benefits of your leadership as a result of what you have done in CHIP. Your landmark study in 1991 opened the floodgates to a lot of these initiatives. That is a tremendous testament. As the only Hispanic on this committee, I want to also say that immigrant children have benefitted as a result of your resolve to make sure that all children are included in the benefits of CHIP and other programs.

Jay, we have a great admiration for you. The best way we can show that admiration is to continue that legacy as we continue to reauthorize CHIP and these other critical programs so that future generations of children in West Virginia and throughout the country will continue to receive the benefits of what you have ultimately achieved for them and for our country.

I have specific questions when we have the witnesses finish their testimony, but I did not want to lose this opportunity to join my colleagues in echoing their sentiments.

Senator ROCKEFELLER. You are a kind man, and I appreciate you. You all are.

Senator Bennet?

OPENING STATEMENT OF HON. MICHAEL F. BENNET,
A U.S. SENATOR FROM COLORADO

Senator BENNET. Thank you, Mr. Chairman. If I could, I would like to take just one minute also to say how grateful I am for your leadership on these issues. I came here having spent almost 5 years of my life being Superintendent of Denver public schools, wondering who in Washington cared about the kids in that school district. I never had any doubt that you did, and my time here has only reaffirmed that.

The *New York Times* columnist, David Brooks, wrote in a different context not that long ago that the future has no lobby in Washington, DC. I think that is a huge part of the problem we have in this city, but he was not exactly right, because the future had a huge lobby in you. I think it is incumbent on all of us in this committee to carry on that work.

So, thank you for everything that you have done, Mr. Chairman.

Senator ROCKEFELLER. Thank you, Senator Bennet, very much. Is it all right if I go to the witnesses? [Laughter.]

Senator WYDEN. I think Senator Portman just joined us.

Senator ROCKEFELLER. Senator Portman, thank you for being here, sir.

Senator PORTMAN. I was here earlier, Mr. Chairman, so I got to hear your opening remarks.

Senator ROCKEFELLER. I know. I saw you.

Senator PORTMAN. That is what I really came for. Forget the witnesses—no. Thank you all for being here. [Laughter.]

OPENING STATEMENT OF HON. ROB PORTMAN,
A U.S. SENATOR FROM OHIO

Senator PORTMAN. A toast to you from our United States Senate bottled water. I enjoyed being a colleague and a friend, and I appreciate your willingness to spend so much of your career focused on this issue of children's health and other important matters, important to West Virginia and to our country.

As you know, you are a neighbor, and so I look forward to staying in touch and look forward to the testimony today, and the opportunity to have this be your final hearing on a topic that is a passion of yours and one that is incredibly important for all of our States. Thank you, Mr. Chairman.

Senator ROCKEFELLER. Thank you, Senator Portman. You are kind. You are very kind.

Now we are going to turn to the witnesses. We have a very good panel.

First, we have Mr. Bruce Lesley. Mr. Lesley is the president of First Focus, which is a bipartisan advocacy organization dedicated to making children and families a priority in Federal policy. Well actually, we will just go right to you.

STATEMENT OF BRUCE D. LESLEY, PRESIDENT,
FIRST FOCUS, WASHINGTON, DC

Mr. LESLEY. Thank you, Chairman Rockefeller, Chairman Wyden, and Senators Enzi, Brown, Casey, Menendez, Schumer, Portman, and Bennet, for having this hearing today about the Children's Health Insurance Program and the positive impact it has had on the lives of millions of children across the country. I would like to start by recognizing Chairman Rockefeller for his lifelong achievements in championing an array of issues that have been critically important to the children of West Virginia and this entire country, including his legacy with respect to CHIP.

Mr. Chairman, as you know, CHIP has been an undeniable bipartisan success story. As those of us who worked on the issue back in 1997 can attest, the lack of health insurance coverage among children was a national tragedy. In fact, one in seven of our Nation's children had no health insurance coverage.

As the National Commission on Children—which was chaired by Senator Rockefeller—found in 1991, perhaps no set of issues moved members of the National Commission on Children more than the wrenching consequences of poor health and limited access to medical care. If this Nation is to succeed in protecting children's health, there must be a major commitment from families, communities, health care providers, employers, and government to meet children's basic health needs and to ensure that all pregnant women and children have access to health care.

Mr. Chairman, that commitment to protecting the health of our Nation's children was answered by Congress in your work in a bipartisan manner with the passage of CHIP in 1997. Through the leadership of the Senate and this committee, CHIP was created toward the goal of dramatically cutting the number of uninsured children in America.

On that measure, if you look at Figure 1 on page 3 of my testimony, as those numbers indicate, CHIP has been an incredible success story, as the uninsured rate for our Nation's children has been cut in half—from 14 percent in 1997 to just 7 percent in 2012—while the uninsured rates for adults during that period increased.

In addition to the fact that CHIP is a national success story, it is also bipartisan. One of the hallmarks of CHIP has been the willingness of leaders on both sides of the aisle—you noted this in your work with Senators Hatch, Kennedy, Grassley, and others on this committee—to work together to increase the enrollment of children.

CHIP is also a public/private partnership. CHIP gives States discretion in working with their providers and insurance plans to set premiums, cost-sharing benefits, income eligibility levels, and provider networks for children and pregnant women, rather than having a one-size-fits-all Federal standard.

CHIP is also child-focused. By definition, CHIP is child-focused, and that has been a critical factor in its success for children. CHIP provider networks have been built and improved over the 17 years of its history in every single State, and they meet specific pediatric quality standards that address the unique development and health care needs of children.

CHIP has also been successful in reducing health disparities. In addition to the coverage improvements, a study published by the National Institutes of Health found that CHIP coverage has been critically important and successful in reducing disparities in access to care measures and quality of care.

CHIP is also overwhelmingly popular with the American people. In poll after poll, CHIP has remained popular with the public. The American Viewpoint Poll this past May found that voters support extending CHIP by a wide margin of 74 to 14 percent, and by more than a 3½ to 1 margin even among Tea Party supporters. No matter the political, ethnic, gender, age, or geographic breakdown, CHIP is overwhelmingly popular.

Unfortunately, CHIP's 8 million children are at risk. Although CHIP celebrates its 17th birthday this year and has achieved a remarkable record of success, funding for the program expires on September 30, 2015, and there is some urgency to addressing this issue as soon as possible, because States are beginning their budget preparations now and are facing uncertainty about how to handle CHIP beginning in October 2015.

The consequences of CHIP expiring would spell disaster for more than 8 million children. The reasons are, first, due to what is referred to as the kid glitch in the Affordable Care Act or ACA. It is estimated that up to 2 million children could lose coverage entirely if CHIP were to expire. Second, as a recent First Focus study highlights, rural children will be at the greatest risk if CHIP expires, because children in rural communities would disproportionately lose their health coverage. Last, even for the children who would be able to transition to the Affordable Care Act exchange plans or marketplace, a report by Wakely Consulting Group found that children in every single State would be left with fewer benefits and far-higher cost sharing if they lost CHIP coverage.

Therefore, we urge Congress to, first and foremost, adopt a 4-year extension of CHIP funding through 2019. This would rightfully align the funding with the program's reauthorization date. We urge the Congress to pass such an extension during the lame duck session, as there is some urgency to this.

In addition, we would urge the extension of outreach and enrollment grants, the pediatric quality standards, and Express Lane Eligibility, which expires in March 2015, so that we continue to make progress toward the goal of covering all children.

In closing, I would like to, once again, thank Chairman Rockefeller and the members of this committee for holding this important hearing about children's health. This committee has always provided the leadership on CHIP, and we look forward to working with you toward its extension.

I would also like to personally recognize and thank Chairman Rockefeller—during my time on this committee, my 12 years on the Hill, 10 years in the Senate—for his outstanding career as a champion for our Nation's most vulnerable citizens, its children. We appreciate all that you have done over the years for kids. Thank you very much.

Senator ROCKEFELLER. Thank you, sir, very, very much.

[The prepared statement of Mr. Lesley appears in the appendix.]

Senator ROCKEFELLER. Dr. James Perrin is a primary care pediatrician and president of the American Academy of Pediatrics. In addition to being a lifelong advocate for improving children's health, he is a former professor of pediatrics at Harvard and director of the division of pediatrics at Massachusetts General Hospital.

We welcome you, sir.

STATEMENT OF JAMES M. PERRIN, M.D., FAAP, PRESIDENT, AMERICAN ACADEMY OF PEDIATRICS, ELK GROVE VILLAGE, IL

Dr. PERRIN. Thank you, Senator Rockefeller. I am Jim Perrin, and I join you today on behalf of the 62,000 primary care pediatricians, pediatric subspecialists, and pediatric surgeons at the Academy of Pediatrics. I am in Massachusetts and currently president of the Academy.

Let me start by thanking you and your colleagues here for the opportunity to testify before the subcommittee regarding the CHIP program. Strongly bipartisan in its beginning and strongly bipartisan today, CHIP has developed into a critical program that finances health coverage for over 8 million children across the country and has improved three important aspects of children's health. One is access to coverage, second is utilization of those services, and third is the population health of millions of children who have benefitted from this program.

Coverage is important for a number of reasons, and I think we know that. Uninsured children are three times more likely than children with insurance to lack access to needed medications and five times more likely to have an unmet need for medical care. And a just-released report from the CDC shows that uninsured children receive substantially lower rates of preventative services.

We all know that children are different from adults, and the needs of children—in the sense of their health care needs, in the context of their developmental needs over time, the changing manifestations of disease at different times in the child's life, and the different response to treatments—all require children-specific kinds of benefits. That is exactly what the Children's Health Insurance Program has provided to us.

Most children are healthy, so the epidemiology of pediatric disease really does differ from that of the adult population. Care for all children is marked by adequate immunization and other preventative services. Pediatricians really think prevention is a critical aspect of what we do. Nevertheless, we also have large and increasing numbers of children with chronic health conditions that affect their health and development and require specific care to generate, maintain, and restore age-appropriate functioning to maximize their potential—another area of prevention that is incredibly important.

Children also are different because they represent the most economically, ethnically, and racially diverse population in the United States, with very high rates of childhood poverty. The resulting health care disparities that relate to poverty really increase the risk of adverse outcomes. So these differences between children and adults require distinct and specific services for infants, children, and adolescents that do emphasize the preventative notion.

Now, we have not achieved coverage of these services for every child in the United States, but we should all be proud and thankful for the vast strides we have made since SCHIP was established, as Bruce just reminded us. Today CHIP is critical in helping to ensure that no child falls through the cracks and that the vast majority of U.S. children have access to high-quality affordable health insurance. In fact, even with persistent poverty among children, since

SCHIP's enactment in 1997, the number of uninsured children has been cut in half while, on the other hand, the number of uninsured adults rose significantly.

So the reauthorization in 2009 included several improvements, such as better age-appropriate health benefits; coverage of dental, mental health, and substance abuse services to the same extent as medical and surgical treatments; and a strong Federal investment for the first time ever in children's health care quality improvement.

The Academy urges Congress to fully fund CHIP through at least 2019, and to do so during this Congress, for a host of reasons. Pediatricians are intimately familiar. We work closely with our friends in Alabama, for example, with the interaction between the Federal and State Governments related to Medicaid and CHIP.

States, in particular, need the time to plan and to have an understanding of what the Federal Government will do in order to make wise budgetary decisions. Children and families need the stability that a medical home offers, consistent rules regarding what their insurance covers and the managed care company with which they will interact, and the peace of mind, which we heard about earlier, that quality, affordable health care offers. Pediatricians need to know that they will be able to operate their practices with a reliable payer as well, so that they can keep the medical home open to as many publically insured families as possible.

CHIP has made important contributions to the advancement of health care delivery to near-poor children in recent years and has the potential to accomplish more in the years to come. The Academy specifically offers the following recommendations to strengthen the CHIP program for children: first, to fully fund the program through 2019; to expand awareness of CHIP among eligible families (and indeed, the movement towards exchange plans has helped enroll people in CHIP, which we are very excited about); to facilitate enrollment in CHIP for eligible children; to maximize comprehensive coverage and affordability for children whose care is financed by CHIP; to enhance and continue the very important quality measurement funding and quality improvement funding in the CHIPRA Act; and to ensure adequate payment for physicians who care for CHIP patients.

Children and pediatricians owe tremendous thanks to you, Chairman Rockefeller, to Senator Hatch, Senator Wyden, Senator Roberts, and the other Senators who are here and have been here today, for your bipartisan leadership and working to keep CHIP strong for children. America's pediatricians urge Congress to support your efforts and others in Congress to continue CHIP's success for at least 4 more years.

Thank you very much.

Senator ROCKEFELLER. Thank you, sir, very much.

[The prepared statement of Dr. Perrin appears in the appendix.]

Senator ROCKEFELLER. Ms. Cathy Caldwell is the Director of the Bureau of Children's Health Insurance in the State of Alabama at its Department of Public Health.

You head up the CHIP program, All Kids. I think that is what it is called. It provides coverage to about 85,000 children. I am interested in what you have to say, and I will have follow-up questions as to the disruption in State government and planning, generally.

We welcome you here very much.

STATEMENT OF CATHY CALDWELL, DIRECTOR, BUREAU OF CHILDREN'S HEALTH INSURANCE, ALABAMA DEPARTMENT OF PUBLIC HEALTH, MONTGOMERY, AL

Ms. CALDWELL. Chairman Rockefeller, Chairman Wyden, Ranking Member Roberts, Ranking Member Hatch, Senator Enzi, and distinguished members of the committee, I thank you for allowing me to speak.

In Alabama, more than 82,000 children are currently enrolled in CHIP. More than 56,000 are enrolled in All Kids, which is a separate, stand-alone program, and 26,000 enrollees receive services through the Medicaid program. I am here to ask you to extend CHIP funding beyond fiscal year 2015. Extension is critically needed to continue providing quality care for our children.

CHIP is a successful program. For example, 90 percent of our enrollees have at least one visit with a primary-care physician annually, and our immunization rate for 2-year-olds exceeds 70 percent. We encourage families to seek preventive care over emergency care, and we have seen success. For instance, only 10 percent of our enrollees with asthma have an asthma-related trip to the emergency room, and more than 80 percent of our enrollees with diabetes have an annual A1c test. We provide an enhanced, child-based dental benefit, and more than 60 percent of our enrollees receive a dental visit within 90 days of enrollment.

We also take care of very sick children. Last year alone, we provided coverage to 33 children who have leukemia. In May, we covered a sound processor for a cochlear implant for a 14-year-old boy with hearing loss, allowing him to hear clearly. In June, we enrolled a 7-year-old uninsured child hospitalized with pneumonia, and we enrolled a 13-year-old uninsured girl with cystic fibrosis who had not been able to buy her medication.

These stories are not unique. We hear them every day. We are passionate about taking care of these children who, without CHIP, likely would be uninsured and unable to get the care they need. Across the Nation, there are 8 million children enrolled and depending on an extension of CHIP funding.

While some CHIP children may have access to coverage through an employer group, the cost of dependent coverage may be cost-prohibitive for the family. In addition, employer-sponsored or marketplace coverage may have higher deductibles, premiums, and co-pays than CHIP, leaving even insured children without access to the services and medications they need.

CHIP is a very efficient program. In Alabama, our administrative cost is less than 6 percent of the total cost of our program. We process 99 percent of applications within 10 days, and 90 percent of our claims are processed within 14 days, ensuring our providers are paid timely.

It is important that a decision to extend CHIP funding be made soon. States are developing budgets for fiscal year 2016 now. States cannot make adequate plans with the uncertainty of continued funding for CHIP. Families are relying on you to make this decision soon. The uncertainty of CHIP continuation is stressful for them. The uncertainty also is stressful for employees of these programs. We may lose our very best employees because of this uncertainty. They may seek employment elsewhere.

Before CHIP, the un-insurance rate for children in Alabama was 15 percent. In 2013, the un-insurance rate for Alabama was 8.2 percent. CHIP is successful. It was started to give kids access to health insurance. There is still a need for CHIP. Through CHIP, you have provided routine and life-saving care to our kids.

I ask you to extend funding for the Children's Health Insurance Program, and to do it soon.

Thank you again, chairmen, ranking members, and distinguished members of the committee, for allowing me to speak.

Senator ROCKEFELLER. Thank you very, very much, Ms. Caldwell.

[The prepared statement of Ms. Caldwell appears in the appendix.]

Senator ROCKEFELLER. Finally, we have Dr. Douglas Holtz-Eakin, who is the president of the American Action Forum and is former Director of the Congressional Budget Office, which is fairly awesome. He is an acclaimed expert on fiscal policy matters who has held positions at multiple conservative think tanks and congressional fiscal commissions.

We welcome you.

STATEMENT OF DOUGLAS HOLTZ-EAKIN, Ph.D., PRESIDENT, AMERICAN ACTION FORUM, WASHINGTON, DC

Dr. HOLTZ-EAKIN. Thank you, Mr. Chairman, Senator Portman, and Senator Casey. It is a privilege to be here today to talk about this topic. I have a longer statement I have submitted for the record.

In these opening remarks, I have three simple points, the first of which is that inaction looks very problematic, to say the least. The second is that the ACA has changed the landscape and that, going forward, the CHIP program should likely be modified to reflect that changed landscape. And three, the CHIP Program has a lot of features which have proven to be very, very successful and durable and should be kept in the program as those modifications take place. Let me elaborate a little bit on that.

There are three key aspects of the budgetary situation that really stand out. The first has been noted: funding ends after 2015. The second is that the ACA has a requirement of a Maintenance of Effort for States in their CHIP programs through 2019. The third is that the CBO baseline funding for the program is only $5.7 billion for the years after 2015.

The first two of those features mean that if nothing is done, States are going to be in significant budgetary trouble. They have an obligation to continue the programs, and, depending on how they have done it—as a stand-alone, Medicaid expansion, or a partnership—they are going to face deficits of one type or another. The third feature means that if the Congress chooses to go forward with a program that is anything like the size of the current one, it is going to need more budgetary resources. So something is going to have to give, and action will be required.

The second key point is that the ACA has really changed the landscape. First and foremost, the exchange subsidies are now available for those at 138 percent of the Federal poverty line, up to 400 percent, overlapping with the traditional CHIP eligibility. Indeed, when the ACA was first passed, I thought we would not need a CHIP program anymore. I think many people thought that, but it turns out that is just not true.

As has been mentioned, there is this family glitch in the ACA where employers can satisfy their obligation under the mandate by offering the employee coverage, but not family coverage, and, as a result, he or she will have a family and children who are not eligible for subsidies in the exchanges. Our estimate at the American Action Forum is that there are about 1.6 million children in CHIP right now who will find themselves in that situation. There are another 645,000 who are uninsured at the moment who will find themselves in that situation. That is a population that CHIP traditionally has covered and should cover going forward.

It is also true that, depending on how States have done it, some of those who use CHIP money to expand Medicaid are going to have insufficient funding if nothing is done. That is another almost 500,000 children at risk. That brings a targeted population of about 2.7 million that have a real need for a CHIP program, despite the passage of the ACA.

The third thing I would mention is, simply, in trying to remodel the program for the future, hold on to some things that have been successful. The bipartisanship has been mentioned in the past, and I want to echo that. When I was CBO Director, working on CHIP was a relative pleasure. Very few Senators yelled at me. [Laughter.]

It would be wonderful to see that tradition continued. It also is a program that, in part, got that success because it was narrowly targeted. It is not an open-ended entitlement. Congress thought hard about who belonged in there and provided the funds for that.

Right now, if we did the 2.7 million that I mentioned, that would be under $6 billion a year, based on a rough estimate of ours. Or you could continue the program in its current incarnation, and that would be, maybe, $20 billion in 2016. So there is a real range of funding amounts that would come out of trying to figure out the population that the Congress wants to cover.

And the last thing is the great success at letting the States manage this in a flexible fashion. I think that has been a hallmark of the CHIP program and something that both the committee and the Congress should think about as they build a CHIP program for the future.

In closing, just let me add my voice to those congratulating you on an outstanding record of public service and say it is a privilege to be here today and to answer your questions. Thank you.

Senator ROCKEFELLER. Thank you, sir, very, very much.

[The prepared statement of Dr. Holtz-Eakin appears in the appendix.]

Senator ROCKEFELLER. I am interested in the children who still have to be reached out to, in the Alabamas and West Virginias and Pennsylvanias and Ohios, et cetera. There are still so many.

Let us just take Alabama. I am going to ask you a two-part question, Ms. Caldwell. The business of outreach is often not the question of the State, or a group of doctors, or citizen action groups reaching out. It is getting past the parents and getting the parents to buy into the program.

Having health insurance is a fabulous thing. So is having an education. But you and I both know that in West Virginia and in Alabama, with bus service often scanty for most rural areas, parents will withhold the child going to school, saying, if you go to school, it is not going to get you anywhere anyway, so stay home and let us work on the garden.

In other words, that is a problem. That is a problem. It is not something that the parents faced—they had education, they did not have education—but, with respect to their children, they just think differently, and they think in terms of convenience. From their real-world perspective, getting an education does not seem to prove that it is going to turn into a lot of dollars.

So, one, how do you go about outreach in Alabama, or how should we do it generally? And second, this whole question of disruption is really hard for me. I will just put it this way: it is a really popular program. But it was, I think, Senator Casey, Senator Portman, the last amendment at 2 o'clock in the morning on the—what was it?—8-day markup we had on the Affordable Care Act. It was the last amendment, and the presiding person at that session turned to me—I was sitting at his side—and asked me not to bring up CHIP. I did not ask him what his reasons were. I just said that I was not going to follow those instructions. I was going to bring it up, and it did pass.

We talk about bipartisanship, how people agree on things, but then things can come up, either placement or disposition of time, or the mood of the leadership, or whatever it is. Politics can come into it. So you cannot always count on something which has been bipartisan to continue to be bipartisan. I hope we can. All I know is, I am fighting really hard, knowing that there are people who do not want to see this happen.

So could you address the question of outreach and also the question of disruption and why having multiple ways of going at the CHIP program is comforting to your Governor and to Governors throughout the United States?

Ms. CALDWELL. I would love to, and I too would like to add my thanks for your service, particularly to the children of our country and your great CHIP Director, Sharon Carte. She is one of my very special colleagues and friends, and she is retiring in the near future as well, but she has just worked so hard for the children of West Virginia.

So, outreach—I think Alabama has some best practices around previous outreach. We had always conducted a lot of outreach targeted to all uninsured children in our State. The higher percentage of those were Medicaid-eligible, as is seen in every other State. The bulk of the uninsured children in our country are actually Medicaid-eligible, then a smaller proportion are CHIP-eligible.

Approximately 2½ years ago, we stopped outreach in Alabama because of State budget problems. There just was not sufficient State funding for us to continue the outreach we were doing. Particularly, we could not really afford for our program to grow at the rate it had been growing, so we stopped outreach. Nobody was particularly happy with that. It was just the reality of funding.

What we found through all of the years we were doing outreach is that it is important to keep the message out there continuously, because families find themselves in different situations. If your children have always been privately insured, you may tend to not pay that much attention to Medicaid or CHIP. Then all of a sudden, there may be a job loss, and the family needs these programs.

So we found that we needed to be out there telling families what Medicaid was, what CHIP was, really targeting all of the uninsured children. We have always partnered with all of our provider groups. The Alabama chapter of the American Academy of Pediatrics is just one of our number one partners.

So, even though the State has not conducted organized outreach in the last few years, our community partners have absolutely stepped up. So, in getting the word out, getting the information out to all of our partners, we certainly have always partnered very closely with school nurses and other school staff. So just being everywhere and targeting all of the uninsured children I think is great, and I certainly have hated that we have stopped outreach in Alabama. Hopefully it will come back before too long.

As far as the disruption, if funding is not continued for CHIP, it is going to be a nightmare. It is going to be a nightmare on many levels. Certainly on the State level, we are already dealing with issues related to the uncertainty of CHIP funding. We are preparing our 2016 budget right now. What I have asked my staff to do is to prepare a budget assuming we are funded and assuming the current match rate, because, as you know, the law calls for an increase of 23 percentage points for the Federal match rate for CHIP beginning in 2016. That would be 100-percent Federal funding for Alabama.

That versus no continuation of funding which—I see a zero. That is two opposite ends of the spectrum, zero funding versus 100-percent Federal funding. So we are picking something in the middle of the road.

That is just my guidance to my staff. Now, as far as how the legislature will view funding the program under this uncertainty, I think we will just have to wait and see. We have families already getting stressed. We have staff already getting stressed.

When we enroll a child in CHIP, we award them 12 months of continuous coverage. So right now, within just a month, when we award a child 12 months of coverage, we are not certain that we can actually guarantee that 12 months of coverage because, by that point in time, if funding has not been extended, possibly the program may not even be in existence. Even that question comes with a huge amount of uncertainty in that, if we knew the program was ending September 2015, we would really need to start ramping down, quit enrolling new kids, possibly start disenrolling current enrollees well before that.

We cannot really do that because, if funding was extended at the last minute, then we would be in violation of Maintenance of Effort. The truth is, there seems to be an awful lot of uncertainty around a State's obligation to the Maintenance of Effort requirement even if funding is not continued.

So those are just a few examples of why I think it would be a nightmare, and the families and the enrolled children are going to be the most affected by far, because just the peace and comfort that enrollment in CHIP has given so many families—this issue just brings about a lot of anxiety. For many of the children who are disenrolled from CHIP, they may find coverage through an employer plan or a marketplace plan, but it is my belief that many will not, and they will go back to being uninsured and not have access to the health services that they need.

Senator ROCKEFELLER. I thank you very, very much, and I apologize to Senator Casey and to Senator Portman that I have overrun my time.

So let us go to Senator Casey, followed by Senator Portman.

Senator CASEY. Mr. Chairman, thank you very much. You have that prerogative anytime, but I guess you have it especially today, to go over your time.

We are grateful for the witnesses' testimony. There is a lot to focus on, but I wanted to focus on the consequences of inaction, the consequences of not moving forward in the direction that we all hope. Mr. Lesley, could you walk through that, just kind of what could happen if we do not act?

Mr. LESLEY. A couple of things, I think, are important. I think my colleague talked about some of the things that her State faces. I would also say that—and I would emphasize Ms. Caldwell's point on what happens to the families and the uncertainty around that and whether the State can commit to a 12-month continuous enrollment.

There is also the issue of the States and their contracts with providers and plans. So how does a State sign a contract with a managed care provider, and how does a managed care provider sign contracts with their provider networks, when there is so much uncertainty about the future of the program, and so much uncertainty about the funding levels, and so much uncertainty about the Maintenance of Effort provision and what all those things mean?

So for us, I think that, even with all the positives about CHIP and all the issues that we found that would happen to kids if they lose insurance, we all know—I have worked up here for 12 years—things happen in Congress, and, if we wait until next year, you would have to look at the vehicles. Would we try to attach it to the SGR? Would there be some sort of budget reconciliation package? There is so much uncertainty around any of that.

In 2007, we know we had this experience: President Bush vetoed the Children's Health Insurance Program at one point, and, as we went through the process, the program actually expired. States were beginning to send out dis-enrollment notices to families. So dis-enrollment notices went out to families in something like more than a dozen States at some point as funding was starting to lapse. Fortunately, Congress stepped in at that point and did an extension. But it was a disaster, because States were looking to fire employees, families were freaking out because they were being told they were about to lose their coverage, and providers did not have any certainty.

One of the things that we know is so important about CHIP in this whole issue of 12-month continuous coverage is that the incentives are to make sure that the kids remain healthy. It really disrupts that, to use Senator Rockefeller's term.

Senator CASEY. I wanted to highlight the chart that you have on page 3 of your testimony and just note it for the record, and not by way of a question, just by way of highlighting it. Based upon your Figure 1 on page 3, if you start in 1997, 14 percent of the children in the country were uninsured. As of 2012, that was cut to 7 percent, so cut in half in that time frame. Obviously, 7 percent is still too high in my judgment. We have work to do, but it is a substantial achievement.

Moving to Dr. Perrin, I guess the point that you made is an oft-repeated maxim, which is that children are not small adults. You cannot just take a health care program and impose that upon the life of a child and expect to get the results we hope for.

I think what your testimony gave us in addition to validating the program from the perspective of the American Academy of Pediatrics—we certainly appreciate that—is a to do list at the end of your testimony: fully funding CHIP through at least 2019, number 1; number 2, expanding awareness; number 3, facilitating enrollment; number 4, maximizing comprehensive coverage and affordability; number 5, enhancing the quality measurement; and number 6, ensuring adequate payments for physicians. So, among other things, that is critically important. I wanted to ask you if there is anything else, any other point you wanted to make from the vantage point of the Academy?

Dr. PERRIN. Senator Casey, thank you. As a native Pennsylvanian, you know a lot about what is going on in CHIP in Pennsylvania. It is an incredibly robust program, really important to the children and families in your great State, so I think it is really critical that we maintain it.

I talked about prevention. I really want to stress that. Obviously we are interested in prevention of coronary artery disease in 50-year-old people as well, but the prevention aspect of what we do with children is so critical to what is going on. We know so much more about the science of development than we did even 10 years ago. We know how much more important it is that we provide early intervention services in the health realm, to really keep kids growing well and successfully.

We know how important it is to our future economy, frankly, that we have a healthy workforce ready to go to work and keep our economy robust. So that preventive aspect is really critical, and it is one of the key aspects of the CHIP program, also of the Medicaid program, by the way, really a critical part of what is going on there.

I will make one other quick comment, which is, we did pass Medicare a couple years ago, in 1965. At that time, a third of elderly Americans lived below the poverty line. Today it is 8 percent, and it is partly because families were kept from health-related bankruptcy.

The CHIP program does some similar things. It does not cut our poverty rate as much as I might like for children, but it surely keeps families able to do things to raise their kids effectively, to be able to let them play sports safely. All those sorts of things are really critical here and, again, because it is a child-specific benefit that really works.

Thank you for that.

Senator CASEY. Thanks, Doctor. Thanks for the plug for our State too.

Senator ROCKEFELLER. Senator Portman?

Senator PORTMAN. Thank you, Mr. Chairman, and thanks to our witnesses. You have given us some good information to be able to prepare for the reauthorization before the end of next year.

I am just a little confused on the cost run. Probably, that is on purpose, but when you look at it, really it is interesting. We have a situation now where we are funding through September 30th of next year, which will be the fiscal year, and yet you have an authorization through 2019. Under the Affordable Care Act, you have a Maintenance of Effort requirement, as I understand it, through 2019, which is really an unfunded mandate, because the funding level is at best uncertain and there is no requirement for funding beyond September 30th of next year.

I also think, on the ACA requirement, it does not have the flexibility you would need, as Ms. Caldwell just talked about in response to the chairman's question.

So, Doug, help us here. As a former Budget Director, what is the situation here in terms of what is in the baseline? What are the assumptions that CBO makes? Is it true that because it is built into the baseline that, say a 2-year extension, for instance, would actually not end up having a cost attached to it because it is assumed that it will be extended? What is the budget situation?

Dr. HOLTZ-EAKIN. The CBO budget numbers reflect what I would label a gimmick in the final passage when it was last funded. In that year, they provided funding for 2015 that consisted of three pieces: a lump sum of about $11 billion, one time, and then two 6-month appropriations at a rate of $2.85 billion for the first and the second half of the year.

CBO, under its rules, when it is asked to extend a program that has not been refunded or reauthorized, continues at the last funding level that the Congress has authorized, so that is $2.85 billion for 6 months, or $5.7 billion per year. That is what is in their baseline.

That clearly will not cover the cost of the existing program if you were to run it out for another 2 years. So the Congress would have to come up with more resources in the process of doing any such extension. And that is a problem for the Congress that was created by the way this was done the last time they passed it.

Senator PORTMAN. You got into this a little bit earlier in your testimony, but do you have an estimate of what that cost increase would be, what the shortfall would be, through a 2-year extension?

Dr. HOLTZ-EAKIN. You are running somewhere between the $5.7 billion you have and the $20 billion you need at the Federal level to fund the program under current law. So you have to come up with another $14 billion a year.

Senator PORTMAN. In terms of the ACA requirement, have you spent any time looking at that?

Dr. HOLTZ-EAKIN. Not in great detail. We know it exists. The CBO, again, in its baseline, does not reflect the higher match rate that the States are counting on, because there is no money to pay that higher match rate, so it simply assumes it does not happen.

Senator PORTMAN. So it goes to a 50-percent match for most States?

Dr. HOLTZ-EAKIN. It just stays at the current match rate, so they do not get the 23 percentage point bump, and it is silent on how the States are supposed to manage that at the other end. The cost of the program still is what it is, but there is no money there.

I am not a legal expert. Just what you do in terms of Maintenance of Effort when it is not funded, I think remains uncertain at best.

Senator PORTMAN. Yes. I see a lot of heads nodding. [Laughter.]

Uncertainty is a concern in Ohio, I know. Every State has a little different approach to this, but one thing we talked about earlier was the fact that States get the opportunity to design these programs so they work best for their children. That flexibility, it seems to me, is the positive thing, actually something that, under Medicaid, we could use some more of. In States like Ohio, where we do have some good innovative ideas, we are looking for the ability to design and administer the program that way.

One question I would have—and I guess, Ms. Caldwell, you would be a good person to answer this—is, could you talk a little about the structure of CHIP as a State block grant and how your State has used that flexibility that you have to provide coverage that is best suited to the children of Alabama?

Ms. CALDWELL. Absolutely, and I think Alabama is a great model. We have a separate stand-alone CHIP program administered in the Alabama Department of Public Health. So we are even in a separate State agency from Medicaid, but we have always worked very, very closely with the Medicaid agency. We have a joint application. We have always had a joint application. Certainly with the Affordable Care Act implementation, we built a joint eligibility system.

When decisions were made about Alabama's CHIP design, there were some very vocal advocates who said, we would like to see a separate stand-alone program, not an expansion of Medicaid, and that is how it was designed. We actually deliver our CHIP benefits through Blue Cross and Blue Shield of Alabama. So our enrollees have access to the exact same network as almost every privately insured individual in our State. I am not saying that would be the best model for every State, but I am saying that it has been a great model in Alabama.

Senator PORTMAN. By the way—I guess this is maybe obvious to all of our witnesses, but, in a State like Ohio, where CHIP is part of our Medicaid program, we take a hit too. So it is not as though, just because you have a stand-alone program, at the end of next year you are going to be in some special situation. All States will have to face this.

I guess if maybe one of our other witnesses could just talk briefly—Mr. Chairman, my time has expired. I am sorry.

Senator ROCKEFELLER. Go ahead.

Senator PORTMAN. Could someone just talk briefly about what impact it would have on States like Ohio where we have it as part of our Medicaid program?

Mr. LESLEY. Senator Portman, thank you. I will speak to that issue and also your previous question too, if that is all right.

So first of all, if CHIP expires, then you would go back to the regular matching rate, and, because of the MOE, you would still be covering the kids. So children would lose coverage, and the State would be out significant financial resources. I believe in Ohio, it would be tens of millions of dollars annually over the course of that period of time. I know with California it would be something like $500 million dollars, for example. So that is a huge impact that it would have on the States.

With respect to the costs, one of the interesting things we know is, when Senator Rockefeller offered his amendment in the Finance Committee to save the CHIP program, one of the things that happened with the CBO scoring was that yes, there was a cost because you were keeping CHIP operating, but there was a savings because the children were not transferring into the Affordable Care Act, for example. The costs were estimated by CBO in the Affordable Care Act to actually be 25 percent greater than the costs in CHIP.

As a result of that, there actually was a scored savings for Senator Rockefeller's amendment, which then allowed for some other improvements to the Affordable Care Act. One of the things we know is that MACPAC asked the CBO to look at this issue, and we understand, secondhand—I have not seen a score on this—that, if you keep CHIP in place without the bump, it actually saves money. With the bump, it actually costs a little bit, but it is within $1 to $5 billion over the 4-year period.

Senator PORTMAN. Thank you. That is very helpful.

Dr. Perrin?

Dr. PERRIN. If I could just make a quick comment, Senator Portman. You, I know, have been very supportive of the really strong network of children's hospitals in Ohio. It is one of the real great activities in Ohio. It is one of your stellar parts of the State——

Senator PORTMAN. I wish my wife were here to hear you say that. She is very involved in one of them.

Dr. PERRIN. I attended medical school in Cleveland, so I was a part of that for a bit of that time. Seriously, it is an incredible benefit to the State and to the children of the State of Ohio.

Those hospitals are highly dependent on Medicaid and CHIP funding. The ability to build the kind of extraordinary programs you have in Cincinnati, Columbus, Youngstown, Dayton, Cleveland, Toledo, et cetera——

Senator PORTMAN. Akron.

Dr. PERRIN. Akron, sorry. Thank you, sir. [Laughter.]

It is really quite amazing. These places would change dramatically without CHIP. There would be cuts in staff. There would be cuts in critical programs to take care of kids with asthma in the State of Ohio, et cetera. There a lot of things that are going on that would change very dramatically in your State if this happened.

Senator PORTMAN. Yes. That is a great point, and we are blessed to have some of the great ones, three of the top ten in the country as rated by at least some rating agencies, including yours, probably.

Thank you, Mr. Chairman.

Senator ROCKEFELLER. Thank you, Senator Portman, very much.

I remember when we got our children tested for sensitivity to ragweed and all kinds of things. We took them out to the University of Cincinnati. It was a wise decision. You did not mention Cincinnati, so I thought I would. [Laughter.]

Senator PORTMAN. Cincinnati Children's Hospital Medical Center, number three in the country based on the latest rating.

Senator ROCKEFELLER. Of course. Of course. [Laughter.]

Just as a follow-up to the question of funding which was addressed, CBO actually has come out with an estimate on what all of this would cost. It is not $20 billion; it is in the area of zero up to $10 billion over that period of 4 years. I only say that, not to argue with you, but simply to say that, in this program, where everything is "maybe, but, if," it is important not to scare people. That was not your purpose, but I just wanted to put that on the record.

To you, Dr. Perrin, the whole question of prevention and health care for children strikes me as so vastly greater than it would have been 10 years ago. I spent a lot of time—every one of my 30 years I have been on the Veterans Committee—working on the Gulf War Syndrome and post-traumatic stress disorder. Actually, there are some remarkable experiments going on with that which are FDA-approved, clinical trials, which show that, by doing certain things, with 2 years of psychotherapy, you can reduce PTSD in veterans—of course, that takes you all the way back to Civil War veterans—by 83 percent. It does not mean it will happen. It is not an approved protocol at this point, but it is on its way.

It is not just adults or veterans who get stressed out and have trauma. Children have extraordinary trauma. You can see that going on now in football. You can see that with kids being molested, kids being beaten up. People have kids who really do not want to have kids, so the family is in turmoil—a mother-in-law does not agree with something, or a father-in-law. Kids can be put down, slammed down really hard at a very early age, and remember it for a long time.

To me, all of that enters into the world of prevention. I remember—and this is a little heretical to say—back in 1989, Senator Jack Danforth, who was a marvelous, marvelous Senator, and I put out the first kind of discussion about end-of-life care, which was immediately slammed down, but we kept bringing it up year after year. It began to be discussed.

I think that sort of discussion is also important for children. What is prevention? It is not just looking for tonsillitis or whatever, giving an immunization shot. There is a lot of psychological aspect to it. I think that this country has opened up enormously to the whole field of mental health, and it is much more tolerant, families are becoming more tolerant, they are becoming more open, about talking about their own situations on that, but much less their children's needs on that.

I would love you to take the field of children and expand it from when you were practicing, let us say 20 years ago, to today's context of horrible television and all kinds of traumas going on in all directions. In what ways are children, do you think, more vulnerable and, therefore, more needy of the kind of prevention that the CHIP program provides?

Dr. PERRIN. Thank you, Mr. Chairman. This is a tremendously important area for how we think as pediatricians. So we are really committed to the notion that a number of folks are working on about making communities places where children can be healthy, where we have a culture of health as part of what our communities are about, rather than a culture of abuse or a culture of violence or a culture of danger where children are not allowed to go outside because they may get shot, et cetera.

We really are working to change that kind of notion. That is the kind of prevention that we really are working on. It is really critical. We know so much more about the science of brain development than we did 15 years ago, and we know that those experiences you just mentioned, about being slammed down and so forth, leave permanent scars, permanent changes in brain architecture and neuroendocrine function of the brain, that really stay there forever and really do limit the child's ability to do the kinds of things that she ought to be able to do as she grows up. So that is where we think of prevention, and we as clinicians are increasingly working on the area of prevention in our collaboration with our other partners in communities to make communities a place of health.

So one of the things that is really exciting about CHIP and Medicaid today is a return to the notion that mental health really belongs in community health. It should not be carved out as it was for probably 25 years, making it such that I could not see a patient in my office with a diagnosis of attention deficit hyperactivity disorder because that was a psychiatric diagnosis. I certainly saw kids with that diagnosis in my office all the time, but I was not allowed to do so under the carve-out arrangements.

Preventative services—identifying children early, identifying family issues early—were very difficult to do because we carved them out of regular health. We considered mental health not regular health. Well, we are bringing it back in.

Senator ROCKEFELLER. You could see it, but you could not do anything about it.

Dr. PERRIN. You could not do anything about it; right. We are bringing that back in. Medicaid and CHIP programs across the Nation, in so many of our States, are moving to reintegration of mental health into primary care.

I will tell you, by the way, clinically, it is incredibly exciting to me. It is so much fun. It is so interesting to work with families to sort of help them understand their strengths, not their weaknesses, to help them build on that, help them think about how to nurture children effectively. That is where we are going, and again, Medicaid and CHIP are moving back in that direction and allowing us to do it. These are really exciting times.

Senator ROCKEFELLER. I am already over my time, and I want to go to Senator Stabenow and, of course, the chairman.

One of the things that always disturbs me—I work a lot with seniors, as the chairman has done for his whole life. One of the things you see is doctors in medical school going into geriatrics, and they are very intense, very determined on that.

When they get into the field, it does not pay as well as some of the other specialties. That was, sort of, one of the things that brought about that ''resource base relative to value scale'' adjustment back in—what was it?—1989 or something like that, where you try to get more parity between primary care physicians and the better-paying specialties.

We found that geriatricians were wandering away from geriatrics and going into other fields for which they were, for the most part, trained. On the contrary is this new emphasis and the excitement which you exhibit, and all of you exhibit, in terms of taking care of children. And they are not little adults, but they are getting a lot of what adults are getting, but have no defenses against it. They just absorb it and so it, sort of, sits in there roiling.

Are you finding that people are more attracted to being pediatricians? Are the rolls growing on that?

Dr. PERRIN. So we have been fortunate in pediatrics in continuing to maintain a pipeline of young people excited about this field and coming into it. I think we are, actually, still doing all right. We are not sure why, because it never pays well compared to all of our other areas in medicine.

Behind me is a young person from the great State of West Virginia who is a young person training in medicine and pediatrics together. These are people who are committed to doing this, and that is what we still recruit. We have not seen a drop-off in people coming into pediatrics. I am really excited to be able to say that.

Now, you know, we still have lots of problems in financing, paying for the kind of care we are trying to provide. Our pediatric subspecialties are not a great pipeline right now. We have a lot of places where we are not getting the people who are kidney specialists, or heart specialists, or blood and guts specialists coming into pediatrics. We need to be working on paying them better, but the Medicaid payment increase is only for primary care. We do not want to treat a child with cystic fibrosis as being worth only two-thirds what a child without cystic fibrosis is.

So we do have some issues to deal with here, but the exciting thing is, it is an incredibly rewarding life. I can say that personally, how wonderful it has been to be a pediatrician in my career. We are still getting wonderfully bright, interesting, committed, passionate people coming into our field. It is different from geriatrics.

Senator ROCKEFELLER. That is great.

Senator Stabenow?

Senator STABENOW. Well, thank you very much, Mr. Chairman. I am so glad I got here before the meeting was over. I apologize, I was——

Senator ROCKEFELLER. It was not going to be over until you got here.

Senator STABENOW. Well, thank you. I was on the floor, as you know, from 3 o'clock to 4 o'clock with other business. I loved when I came into the room that you were talking about mental health, one of the many, many reasons that we are not letting you leave, by the way. You may think you are leaving, but we are not letting you. Senator Wyden, our chairman, has a room, and we are locking you in it. So we are not going to let you leave. [Laughter.]

I really, rather than to ask a question, came specifically, not only to say you need to reauthorize CHIP so that anywhere from 2 million to 4.5 million children who are currently enrolled will not lose their insurance, but also to thank you as the father of CHIP. You are the health care father to millions of children who would not have health care or mental health services, would not have preventative services, without the incredible work that you have done.

I just want to thank you for that. You have not only touched children and families in your beloved West Virginia, but in my beloved Michigan, and Oregon, and everywhere in between. There are generations of adults who will live healthier, happier lives, and parents who have gone to bed at night not having to worry about whether or not the kids got sick, because of your efforts. That is primarily what I wanted to say.

I am also passionate about treating the entire person, the child or adult, and very pleased that, with Chairman Wyden's support, we actually have put in place the beginning of the change here with a first-step pilot project to equalize funding in the community for mental health and public health. I have said over and over again, we need to treat illnesses above the neck the same as below the neck and in a comprehensive way.

So I look forward to working with all of you on that, and to doing everything possible to make sure that CHIP is reauthorized. I think, most importantly today, it is an opportunity to say "thank you" on behalf of tens of millions of people in the country who are living better lives because of Senator Jay Rockefeller. So, thank you.

Senator ROCKEFELLER. I will allow that to stay in the record. [Laughter.]

I want to call on the chairman and then Senator Menendez.

Senator WYDEN. Thank you, Chairman Rockefeller.

Senator Stabenow's comments were, of course, spot-on. I am now trying to figure out how we are going to enforce some of these rules. Senator Stabenow said that Chairman Rockefeller was going to be locked in that room nearby, and I am going to have to discuss that with Sharon. [Laughter.]

I think at this point, Chairman Rockefeller, you have gotten the drift about how strongly our colleagues feel about you.

What I want to do—and today has been a hectic afternoon—is get back to, kind of, one question which I think is pretty key to preserving Chairman Rockefeller's legacy. It deals with what I am sure we are going to get in this debate as it gets fast and furious. I think we are going to get the question with respect to, so we have the ACA, we have the Affordable Care Act, and it expands coverage. So, if we have the Affordable Care Act and it expands coverage, so how come we need this other deal called CHIP?

You and Senator Menendez and everybody else here, you can agree that Chairman Rockefeller is the best thing since night baseball, which has been pretty clearly annunciated here. But people might still say, so, how come we need the CHIP program?

So I want to go through something that I think really outlines it, because it really raises the issue of what I think people in the field have come to call the kid glitch in terms of what might happen, and it actually is sort of a branch of what I am concerned about with respect to health policy generally, which we talked about during the course of the Affordable Care Act, and that is the family glitch. When the free choice voucher that I added to the Affordable Care Act was eliminated, that meant we were going to have a bunch of families falling between the cracks. There is going to be a family glitch.

Let us talk about kids, specifically. Now, my understanding is, for the purposes of determining if a person is eligible for a Federal subsidy to buy health insurance, the IRS bases the calculation off the cost of an individual, rather than a family plan. So we are going to have some real barriers for families who cannot afford to pay the monthly premium for a real family plan. It is going to be more expensive.

So parents may be covered through an employer, though they are unable to afford the cost of insuring their child as well. We will still be in the situation where Medicaid is often not an option, as these families often make too much to qualify, thereby leaving the kids in that no-man's land with respect to being uninsured, generally.

So to me, that would be a real kid glitch which would come about, certainly if CHIP were eliminated, but even if it was reduced substantially. You would have a lot of kids getting hammered by this kind of kid glitch. So I thought of asking this question of two people I have admired for quite some time—Bruce Lesley and Doug Holtz-Eakin. We have others who are very knowledgeable in this field as well.

Mr. Lesley and Dr. Holtz-Eakin, why don't you give me your view about what your take is with respect to the kid glitch. Am I missing something? What are the implications, because it sure looks to me that, certainly if CHIP were even cut back in a significant way, we would have a lot of kids in this no-man's land I have been calling the kid glitch.

Mr. Lesley, Dr. Holtz-Eakin, either of you. I know Senator Menendez has a busy schedule, but I wanted to ask that one question.

Mr. Lesley?

Mr. LESLEY. Yes, sir. Thank you very much, Chairman Wyden.

The kid glitch is absolutely a tremendous problem with respect to the interaction between CHIP and the Affordable Care Act. If CHIP were to expire, we estimate that somewhere in the neighborhood of 2 million kids could lose coverage because of exactly what you described. The family member would be deemed to have affordable coverage, or the employee, but the dependent coverage would not be affordable.

So, even if the family was offered coverage that was maybe like 8 percent of their family income, they would be deemed to have affordable coverage. The family coverage could be as high as 30 percent of family income, which is absolutely unaffordable. Often, we know for a fact that employee coverage is less subsidized for family coverage, and family coverage is 2.7 times the cost of employee-only sponsored coverage.

It is a huge issue. In addition to that, I would note that the Wakely Group report shows that, even for the kids who can migrate and who can get subsidies, we also know, even for them, the cost of coverage, as Chairman Rockefeller talked about earlier, is as much as nine times more expensive in the Affordable Care Act plans than it is in CHIP.

The cost would go up substantially in either setting. The interesting thing to note is that CHIP has been deemed to be a cheaper package than that in the exchange plan. So it does not make a lot of sense that we would move kids from one to the other and leave kids stranded, either uninsured or with more costly out-of-pocket costs and fewer benefits for more money. It would cost the Federal Government more money.

That whole rationale, it leads us to very strongly support the extension of CHIP.

Senator WYDEN. Dr. Holtz-Eakin, is there anything you want to add?

Dr. HOLTZ-EAKIN. As I emphasized in my remarks at the outset, this is a real problem. There is no way around that. Our numbers are a bit higher. We think if you combine the kid glitch and those who get CHIP money devoted to Medicaid expansions, we have 2.7 million children in this category of risk.

The thing I would emphasize for the committee and the Congress is, it is really not a matter of bigger or smaller. CHIP should change. It is in a different environment. There are other vehicles for coverage for other people, and it now resides in an insurance landscape. This is very different than the one in which it was created. It would be beneficial for Congress to address the funding cliff that it faces, but also to think about a CHIP program for the future that fits into this landscape.

Senator WYDEN. Thank you. Thank you, Mr. Chairman.

Senator ROCKEFELLER. Thank you very much.

Senator Menendez?

Senator MENENDEZ. Thank you, Mr. Chairman. I want to talk about two dimensions of CHIP that I think sometimes do not get the attention they deserve. Having heard the last answer about the kid glitch, in my mind it is even more imperative.

Mr. Lesley, in your testimony, you mentioned something that I do not think gets enough attention when discussing CHIP, and that is the impact it has on reducing racial and ethnic disparities. And then there is the success of the *promotora* models of engagement. As a matter of fact, this past Sunday, Nicholas Kristof and Sheryl WuDunn published an article in the *New York Times* highlighting the benefits of early intervention with pregnant women and newborn babies.

Mr. Chairman, I would ask unanimous consent that that article be included in the record.

Senator ROCKEFELLER. So ordered.

[The article appears in the appendix on p. 67.]

Senator MENENDEZ. It highlights a substantial benefit to children and families from early intervention and home visitation. For example, these early intervention programs resulted in a 79-percent reduction in child abuse and neglect, a greater than 50-percent reduction in arrests later in a child's life, and more than

2 fewer years on public assistance programs. So, if you combined those evidence-based programs, they offer nearly a $6 return for every dollar that we invest.

The article also highlights the work of the Nurse-Family Partnership, a group that I have worked with extensively on the Maternal, Infant, and Early Childhood Program, which provides women and children incredibly important and successful services.

So that is a big preface, but what I want to get from you is, can you speak to the impact on children starting at childhood and moving through adolescence when they have access to services like home-visitation alongside other health care services as well?

Mr. LESLEY. Yes. Thank you, Senator Menendez. First and foremost, I would also like to acknowledge an amendment that you offered that was so important in all of this, which is the Child Only Option, which really recognized that children and families often get their coverage separate and apart from their parents. Their parent may be a veteran and have VA care, but the child gets coverage under Kinship Care. Their grandparents may be on Medicare, but they need to get CHIP coverage. That amendment has been huge, and we are really working to try to make it work.

CHIP and Medicaid have had an enormous impact on health disparities. I would note a National Institute of Medicine report in my testimony that talked about some of the impact on disparities. There are also reports from the CDC and ASPE that talk about that.

The coverage differences have been remarkable. We have really shrunk the disparities in coverage. I would note exactly what you said—also noted in Dr. Perrin's testimony and a question I answered—which is this importance of prevention. And NFP has proven that for every dollar you spend, you save enormous amounts of money in long-term savings. It is a medical model where nurses go into the home, and we really believe that it has really facilitated the combination of Medicaid and CHIP in partnership with organizations like NFP.

Also, you mentioned the community health workers or *promotoras* program. When I worked for Senator Bingaman, there was a grant that went to a *promotora* program in Las Cruces, NM, and they had a target of trying to reduce the uninsured rate. I think the uninsured rate in Las Cruces was something around 35 percent, about a third. Literally, these two women got this grant and went from county fair to county fair doing the outreach that Senator Rockefeller was talking about doing—outreach to the community. They had a target of "x," and they actually exceeded it.

The other day we were laughing, because you have 102-percent coverage in Las Cruces now. It was enormously successful, and, not only was it successful in getting coverage to people, but it was also successful in helping families navigate the system. That is another bill you have done in the past, the Patient Navigator, which really helps people navigate the health care system. It was huge for the people in Las Cruces, the combination of those things working together.

Senator MENENDEZ. I appreciate it. Part of our challenge when we score here is that I wish we scored in ways in which we recognize the upside, like the ratio I just described, so that we could factor that in.

If I may, Mr. Chairman, could I ask one other question?

Senator ROCKEFELLER. Please.

Senator MENENDEZ. Dr. Perrin, first of all, I want to thank you and the Academy for the work that you did with me and Senator Enzi on the Autism Care Act earlier this year. I think it is incredibly important.

As you know from that, the State of New Jersey has the highest incidence of children diagnosed with an autism spectrum disorder—one in 49 receiving a diagnosis by the age of 8, compared to one in 68 nationally. Providing resources for children with autism and their families is one of my top priorities, and we are elated that the President signed the Autism Care Act into law, which continues some critical Federal autism programs that were set to expire and a provision that I included in the Affordable Care Act requiring autism services to be included as essential health benefits in all new marketplace insurance plans.

I want to see if you can help me discuss the role that CHIP plays in providing critical behavioral health and autism services to children, and how that help and intervention impacts a child in the autism spectrum disorder in terms of how we maximize whatever their God-given ability might be, and how it affects them as they grow up?

Dr. PERRIN. Thank you, Senator Menendez, and thank you so much for your incredible advocacy for the Autism Care Act. We are really grateful for that. We think that is an incredibly important act for America's children, and it is doing really some extraordinarily important things.

I have been talking about prevention and early intervention all afternoon. I think it is really the critical part of it. We know in an area like autism that it is really critical that we provide services early on, because the brain is still more plastic in a child who is 6 months or a year old to 2 years old than in a child who is really over the hill at age 5—not really, of course, but still, it is really critical to identify kids early and to get them the kind of early intervention services.

You mentioned before, home-visitation as well. It is an area that we have been incredibly supportive of as well, and it is one where we are working very much to integrate and really connect much more actively what is happening in home-visitation and what is happening in community-based pediatrics, because we are working with the same families. We are trying to make sure that the communication is really going well in that context and that we are using that opportunity, again, to build community linkages, link families with resources, and try to help families find the kinds of resources to let them do better.

CHIP is really very important, because the benefits in CHIP are preventive and child-oriented benefits. Yes indeed, we wanted the Affordable Care Act to have similar benefits in the exchange plans, but, as we know well, as the exchange plans have been implemented in large numbers of the States, the benefits for children, especially in behavioral areas and abilitative services, are not really very good.

The CHIP benefits are substantially better in those realms. That is one of the reasons that we are really strongly advocating for the persistence of CHIP here. We will work to make the exchange plans better, no question about it. But right now the benefits for children in exchange plans in general—very much State options as you know—are not great. That is why we are really very committed to CHIP as an important preventive benefit for children.

Senator MENENDEZ. I appreciate that. Thank you, Mr. Chairman.

Senator ROCKEFELLER. Thank you, Senator Menendez.

I have a guilt complex because I have not asked you any questions, Mr. Lesley, but I am going to forgive myself in the interest of everybody else in this room. [Laughter.]

All of us have asked you questions but me. So I apologize.

Let me just say, in bringing this to a conclusion, I am struck by that number. Senator Menendez, you said one in 49 in New Jersey, one in 68 nationally?

Senator MENENDEZ. Yes.

Senator ROCKEFELLER. That is stunning. It has not been reauthorized, CHIP. It is still out there, floating. We are—for reasons that only God could possibly understand—going into recess again in 3 days. The reason for that is actually something which is fairly important in public life, not attractive to many, but important, and that is elections.

That puts terrible pressure on the lame duck session. We are talking about dealing with everything from continuing resolutions, all of the appropriations, what are we going to do about ISIS, and all the rest of it, in a lame duck session forum. That, in turn, will be shaped by whoever wins the Senate. If we keep the Senate, if we do not keep the Senate, that will have its affect.

That, in turn, will have its affect on how CHIP is treated or put in priority. Lots of things are favored and wanted on a bipartisan basis, but they do not make it because the stars and the watches do not align properly for a discussion to be had, for votes to be held, or somebody can hold that up and cannot be talked out of not holding it up.

The Senate has many, many mysterious ways of protecting the rights of the minority and others, but it can fall short in terms of passing legislation. So I want to emphasize that CHIP is not yet included. It is not included. It is out there still. I think it has terrific bipartisan support, but people are so good at picking something in it they do not like, and they do it dramatically, and then it blows up and goes viral.

I worked very hard with Olympia Snowe to start something called the E-Rate to provide connectivity in schools and libraries. I am really happy that we did that, and sometimes I am really unhappy that we did it, because that is now the source of hacking, that is the source of bullying of children, that is the source of all kinds of invasions of privacy, and even shutting down whole hospital systems or power plants. It can have a devastating effect, and often the kids who can do this are less than 15 years old. It is the property and the power that we have given to people for one purpose but that has been used for other purposes.

This is not that kind of a discussion. This is simply a matter of making sure that we get the CHIP program passed, that we get it extended, and that we get it done in what will have to be the lame duck session.

The lame duck session does not sound like anything, but it is. It is a regular session. It is just that some people are there who will not be there, myself included, in the future. I do not want to fool around with CHIP. There just are not that many efforts which are as broadly supported.

I have experienced so many things. Mike Enzi comes from a big coal mining State, but it is a different kind of coal mining State. It is, sort of, digging it out from the earth from the top. West Virginia has underground mining, which is not so much prevalent in Wyoming, and we had a terrible series of explosions there. Senator Enzi came and met with the families, with myself and a few other Senators. You could just see it working on him and within him.

One of his colleagues on the Republican side, Senator Isakson, was one of those who came, and he still carries in his wallet the picture of one of the coal miners who died, which had been given to him by one of the coal miner's children.

So who knows what it is that passes bills and does not pass bills. An endless amount of time helps. We never have that, because the world is in such crisis. Things are happening so disastrously and so unhealthfully. We have to do it as best we can.

CHIP is something we can do. CHIP is something we have to do. I just encourage all of us to think about children, about the problems they face, and about our responsibility to help them navigate their way through those waters.

I thank all of you for your courtesy in coming, and I wish all of us well on the legislation.

The hearing is adjourned.

[Whereupon, at 4:48 p.m., the hearing was concluded.]

APPENDIX

Testimony of Cathy Caldwell

Prepared for oral presentation

United States Senate Committee on Finance

Subcommitee on Health Care

Tuesday, September 16, 2014, 2:30 PM ET

215 Dirksen Senate Office Building

Chairman Rockefeller, Chairman Wyden, Ranking Member Roberts, Ranking Member Hatch and distinguished members of the committee: Thank you for allowing me to speak with you. I am Cathy Caldwell, director of Alabama's Children's Health Insurance Program.

In Alabama, more than 82,000 children are currently enrolled in CHIP: More than 56,000 are enrolled in All Kids, which is a separate, stand-alone program administered by the Alabama Department of Public Health, and 26,000 receive health care services through Medicaid.

I am here to ask you to extend CHIP funding beyond Fiscal Year 2015. Extension is critically needed to continue providing quality care for our children.

CHIP is a successful program. For example, 90 percent of our enrollees have at least one visit with a primary-care physician annually, and our immunization rate for two-year-olds exceeds 70 percent. We encourage families to seek preventive care over emergency care and we have seen success. For instance, only 10 percent of our enrollees with asthma have an asthma-related trip to an emergency room, and more than 80 percent of our enrollees with diabetes have an annual A1c test. We provide an enhanced, child-based dental benefit, and more than 60 percent of children receive a dental visit within 90 days of enrollment.

We also take care of very sick children. Last year alone, we provided coverage to 33 children who have leukemia. In May, we covered a sound processor for a cochlear implant for a 14-year-old boy with hearing loss, allowing him to hear clearly. In June, we enrolled a seven-year-old uninsured child hospitalized with pneumonia and we enrolled a 13-year-old uninsured girl with cystic fibrosis who had not been able to buy medication. These stories are not unique. We hear them every day. We are passionate about taking care of these children who, without

CHIP, likely would be uninsured and unable to get the care they need. Across the nation, there are 5.8 million children enrolled and depending on an extension of CHIP funding.

While some CHIP children may have access to coverage through an employer group, the cost of dependent coverage may be cost-prohibitive for the family. In addition, employer-sponsored or Marketplace coverage may have higher deductibles, premiums and co-pays than CHIP, leaving even insured children without access to the services and medications they need.

CHIP is a very efficient program. In Alabama, our administrative cost is less than 6 percent of our total cost. We process 99 percent of applications within 10 days and 90 percent of our claims are processed within 14 days, ensuring our providers are paid timely.

It is important that a decision to extend CHIP funding be made soon. States are developing budgets for Fiscal Year 2016 now. States cannot make adequate plans with the uncertainty of continued funding for CHIP. Families are relying on you to make this decision soon. The uncertainty of CHIP continuation is stressful for them. The uncertainty also is stressful for employees of these programs. We may lose our best employees because of this uncertainty. They may seek employment elsewhere.

Before CHIP, the uninsured rate for children in Alabama was 15 percent. In 2013, the uninsured rate for children in Alabama was 8.2 percent.

CHIP is successful. It was started to give kids access to health insurance. There is still a need for CHIP. Through CHIP, you have provided routine and life-saving care to our kids.

I ask you to extend funding for the Children's Health Insurance Program, and to do it soon.

Thank you again chairmen, ranking members and distinguished members of this committee for allowing me to speak to you.

United States Senate Subcommittee on Health
Public Hearing
"The Children's Health Insurance Program: Protecting America's Children and Families"
September 16, 2014

Responses to Questions for the Record From Cathy Caldwell

<u>Senate Finance Committee Chairman Wyden:</u>

As Chairman of the Senate Finance Committee, I am keenly aware of the importance of providing as much certainty as possible when it comes to essential financing and budgeting issues. I'm particularly interested in ensuring Congressional decisions around CHIP financing do not negatively impact children as states engage in CHIP budgeting and planning activities.

Question #1: Director Caldwell, during your testimony, you stated it is important a decision to extend CHIP funding be made soon and that states cannot make adequate plans with the uncertainty of continued funding. Can you provide additional information on the state budget and planning process and how the uncertainty around CHIP funding is affecting the state government as well as children and families?

Answer: Alabama's fiscal year is October 1–September 30. We are currently preparing our CHIP budget request for FY 2016, which will begin October 1, 2015. Included in the Affordable Care Act is an increase in the match rate for CHIP up to 23 percentage points beginning October 1, 2015, which results in 100 percent federal funding for Alabama's program. The uncertainty of funding; whether there will be funding, and, if so at what state match rate makes it difficult to competently articulate the budget request. If the request reflects 100 percent federal funding, (no state funding), and state funding was later needed, it would likely be impossible to find those state dollars after the budget is approved. The budget request will be presented to the Governor who will present a state budget to the legislature. The Alabama legislature will convene in March. It is anticipated that many final agency allocations will be well below requests.

Alabama's CHIP staff is currently working to accurately predict the level of federal funds that will be available at the end of this fiscal year. This information is needed to determine at what month the program will need to shut down if funding is not extended. The program has to accurately predict claims that have been incurred but not billed to ensure enough funds are available to cover these costs. These calculations are complex and a great amount of staff time is being devoted to this effort. Currently, CHIP provides 12 months of continuous coverage and the program is approving children for 12 months coverage, which means right now the program is awarding coverage for which there may not be funding. Because of the Maintenance of Effort requirement, the program is unable to alter this process at this time. The uncertainty is difficult and plans are being drafted along with a timeline for preparation for a shutdown of the program if it becomes necessary.

Additionally, advocacy and professional groups have begun their efforts to encourage Congressional support of the extension and are currently educating the medical community and families. As the awareness increases, so does the anxiety of families, providers, and staff about the potential loss of the program.

<u>Health Subcommittee Chairman Rockefeller:</u>

IMPACT OF CHIP FUNDING EXPIRATION

If CHIP funding expires, children will not simply just transition into other forms of coverage. The dismantling of CHIP will be a messy process—making children's coverage unaffordable for many families. From where I'm sitting, I just don't understand how states are going to find a way to transition over 5.3 million children enrolled in separate CHIP programs into other forms of health insurance, while maintaining affordable coverage for families that rely on CHIP for child-specific care.

Question #1: Director Caldwell, can you articulate what the consequences would be for families and state governments if Congress does not extend CHIP funding?

Answer: Currently, CHIP provides 12 months of continuous coverage and the program is approving children for 12 months coverage, which means right now the program is awarding coverage for which there may not be funding. If the program is not funded, the families will need advance notice to allow them time to seek other coverage for their children. There is concern that not only will some children have a change of coverage, but many children may become uninsured. Children may have access to employer sponsored coverage; however, the family premiums are unaffordable. These children may not be eligible for premium tax credits through the marketplace. There will also be children in the middle of their course of treatment, and there will need to be ample time to allow coordination for these children as they transition to other provider networks. For example, a child going through chemotherapy or in a traumatic brain injury rehab does not need to be suddenly transitioned to a different provider because they have transitioned to a new network.

Beyond concern that children may become uninsured and lack care, the employees administering the program may also become unemployed.

Opening Statement
Senate Finance Subcommittee Hearing
The Children's Health Insurance Program: Protecting
America's Children and Families

Senator Michael B. Enzi

September 16, 2014

Mr. Chairman, thank you for holding this hearing on an important issue in health care. We may not always agree on every health care bill that comes before us, but we certainly agree that the health of our young people vitally important to our health as a nation. You have made children's health a cornerstone of your career here in the Senate, and I applaud your efforts in raising the profile of this issue.

I am hopeful that we can have a very positive dialogue about the path forward for CHIP. I think one of the program's greatest strengths is flexibility to the states. We need to focus our efforts here on identifying core mission of the program in a way that builds on the good work that many states are doing, and which serves the population that truly needs help.

I thank your witnesses for being here today to share your perspectives on the program.

The Children's Health Insurance Program:
Status and Outlook

The United States Senate Committee on Finance
Subcommittee on Health

Doug Holtz-Eakin, President*
American Action Forum

September 16, 2014

*The views expressed here are my own and not those of the American Action Forum, the Partnership for the Future of Medicare, or the Center for Health and Economy. I thank Angela Boothe, Christopher Holt, and Conor Ryan for their assistance.

Chairman Rockefeller, Ranking Member Roberts and members of the subcommittee, thank you for the opportunity to testify on Children's Health Insurance Program (CHIP) today. In my remarks, I will seek to convey three main points about the CHIP program and its future:

- The current budgetary condition of CHIP makes inaction problematic. Instead Congress has an opportunity to review the program and restore it to its original intent.
- A straight funding extension or reauthorization is unwise as CHIP has strayed from its initial targeted design and because of changes forced by the Affordable Care Act (ACA).
- Reauthorization should retain features of the CHIP program that have made it successful, and the program should again be targeted on a specific population.

I will discuss each of these in turn. First, however, some background on the program will be helpful.

Background

Research shows that a lack of health insurance causes unmet medical needs and delays in care for children,[1] demonstrating the need for children to have access to health care services. CHIP is one avenue through which children can gain health insurance in families that may not otherwise be able to provide coverage. However, CHIP should be viewed in the context of the other options available, and with the other federally funded programs that now cover the same population.

CHIP was established by the Balanced Budget Act of 1997, through a bipartisan legislative process that addressed the policy concerns of both sides of the aisle. The program was designed as a block grant, calculating a percentage of funding from the federal government to states based on their CHIP eligible populations. Just as with the Medicaid program, states are provided with federal matching funds—known as the Federal Medical Assistance Percentage (FMAP)—and states receive higher matching rates for CHIP, with the federal government covering about 71 percent of the programs' costs on average. However, as CHIP is an *allotment* to states it does not have an open ended funding stream.[2] CHIP often includes personal responsibility provisions in its financing, incorporating cost-sharing mechanisms for families with higher incomes.

CHIP covered 6 million children as of December 2013.[3] Eligibility rules vary by state, ranging from 138 percent of the Federal Poverty Level (FPL) up to 405 percent FPL depending on the program decisions made by each state.[4] Most states cover above 200 percent FPL, and can receive the increased federal match offered by CHIP up to 300 percent FPL.[5] Some families are subject to cost sharing requirements including monthly premiums and co-pays, depending on the state and the family's financial status. Benefits vary by state but CHIP is known to be a robust program, offering rich benefits and extensive provider networks.

CHIP is a joint federal-state partnership program, and every state participates. Each state has some flexibility over the administrative structure and benefit requirements for their program. The options for structuring the program include the following: a completely separate CHIP program, an expansion of the state's Medicaid program, or a CHIP-Medicaid partnership. Fifteen states run standalone programs, eight states[6] implement the program through an expansion of Medicaid, and twenty eight states opt for a partnership model.[7]

States that choose to provide CHIP through a stand-alone program can offer a variety of benefits to children. States have the option of providing coverage mirroring Medicaid benefits, using the benefits for a state employee plan, or can even choose an HMO benchmark plan. If states use CHIP funding to expand Medicaid coverage, then Medicaid benefit rules apply and children in CHIP will receive Medicaid benefits. For the majority of states, the choice of a partnership model allows states to provide a combination of the two above approaches.[8]

The Budgetary Outlook

The funding for CHIP is not permanent and appropriation of funds must be authorized by Congress. CHIP was originally scheduled for reauthorization in 2007, and was temporarily extended until 2009 when the Children's Health Insurance Program Reauthorization Act (CHIPRA) was passed. CHIPRA was not a straight extension, and made alterations greatly expanding the entitlement program—including increased eligibility levels, patched funding shortfalls, the removal of insurance crowd-out provisions and the institution of bonus payments for states.

As part of the changes in 2009, CHIP spending was only authorized for an additional four years. This temporary extension was put in place as a way of artificially reducing estimated costs of the program. Unfortunately, lawmakers resorted to budget gimmicks during CHIPRA and the ACA.

The authors of the 2009 CHIPRA bill extended funding for CHIP through FY 2013, and the ACA further extended funding through 2015. These temporary extensions create a need for congressional action in the future to fully fund the program in years to come. The ACA extended CHIP, but only left a portion of spending in the baseline after 2015. This mechanism allowed for the bill's apparent cost to decrease without actually saving money on the program. Instead, the program will just require funding authorizations later down the road.

The CBO estimates that the 2014 cost of covering these children is $10 billion, increasing to $11 billion in 2015.[9] CBO does not fully estimate funding levels for the years 2016-2024 because there is no current funding authorization beyond 2015.

Congress divided the 2015 CHIP appropriation into three parts[10]—one large sum at the beginning of the year at $15.4 billion and two smaller sums totaling $5.7 billion, one in the first half and the other in the second half of the year. Because of budget rules, CBO includes in its baseline only the funding in place immediately prior to the scheduled end of funding. Thus the current budget estimate only assumes that annual appropriations of $5.7 billion will continue— an extrapolation of the annualized authorized funding in the latter half of 2015—and that some already appropriated funding will be spent in 2016. CBO estimates that this amount of funding will not be sufficient to cover all the costs of the program. Thanks to some provisions within the ACA, and this budgetary trick, funding will no longer cover the actual cost of the program;

placing states at risk for large budget deficits. Some action must be taken to provide cover for children in need of access to health care and for state budgets.

ACA Challenges and Defining a Tailored Program

As of December 2013, CHIP covered an estimated 6 million children,[11] and the original intent was for CHIP to serve a very specific population.[12] The ACA altered this niche population, changing requirements for covering these children as well as the number of children that still need coverage. For this reason, a straight reauthorization is not the best decision.

The ACA created a requirement for states to maintain current CHIP eligibility levels until 2019; this is known as the Maintenance of Effort (MOE) requirement. Though states are required to maintain their current eligibility levels until 2019, the ACA only provides funding for CHIP through September of 2015. In the absence of congressional action, states could be required to continue a partnership program without their federal partner for up to four years. Depending on a state's program structure, the MOE liability could leave states covering 100 percent of CHIP funding, or states' funding could be reduced to Medicaid levels, creating large budget deficits at the state level. Even with continued federal funding, the Government Accountability Office estimates that half of all states will scale back CHIP in 2020—the first year where these restrictions are lifted.[13] This is especially of concern for states that used CHIP to fund Medicaid coverage for children up to the minimum eligibility level for premium tax credits in the exchange. Without CHIP funding, AAF estimates[14] that states will be responsible for covering 460 thousand children at a lower matching rate who would otherwise lose access to health insurance coverage.

This scale back of the program will be due in part to another issue within the ACA: the overlapping coverage options available to CHIP families. The ACA's insurance Exchanges exist in every state, and provide subsidies for health insurance premiums to families between 138 and 400 percent FPL—largely the same population as CHIP. This redundancy would lead one to assume the CHIP program is no longer needed because entire families can participate in a plan offered through and subsidized by the insurance Exchange in their state that has been advertised as comprehensive, affordable health care coverage. Unfortunately this is not the case for many children, in part due to what has become known as the family glitch.

Though the ACA mandates that employers offer affordable coverage for their employees, the administration has interpreted this requirement as applying only to the employee, and not extending the same benefits to members of the employee's family.[15] If an employee is offered affordable individual coverage through their place of work, then they *and* their family are no longer eligible for subsidized insurance in the Exchange.

The American Action Forum has estimated[16] that, if CHIP funding is not continued, the family glitch could result in as many as 2.28 million children losing access to health insurance coverage. Of those 2.28 million children, 1.6 million are currently enrolled in CHIP and could fall into this loophole, losing their CHIP coverage, and another 645 thousand are currently uninsured but are CHIP eligible and would lose access to coverage. The coverage gap created by the family glitch and the implications for state Medicaid budgets show how the ACA expanded coverage to new populations, while leaving up to 2.7 million children that have been promised coverage in potential limbo. The following graphic shows the possible coverage options for families and children in CHIP:

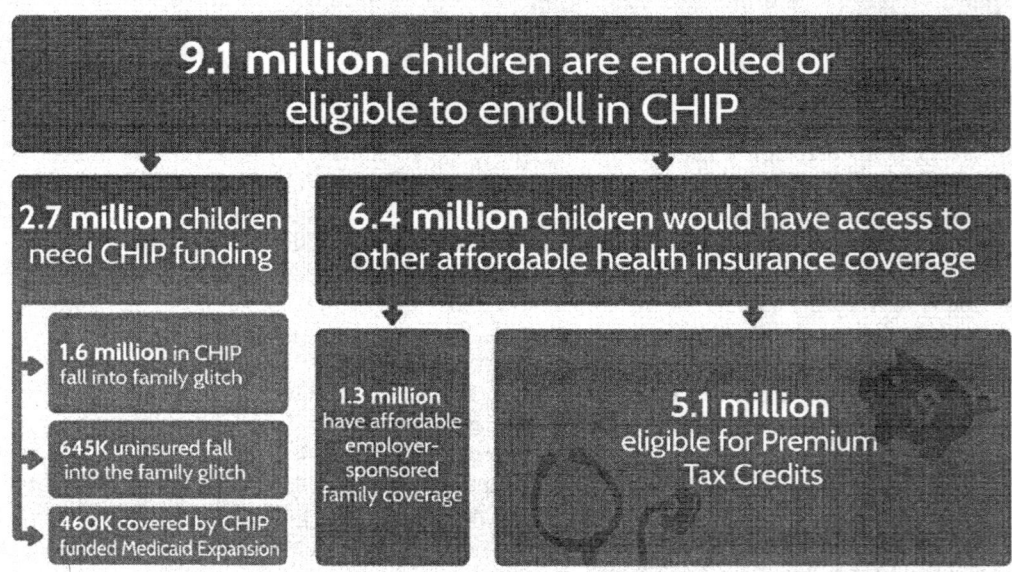

How does CHIP re-authorization affect children's health insurance coverage?

What is CHIP?

The Children's Health Insurance Program was created in 1997 to cover children whose families' income was too high to qualify for Medicaid but couldn't afford insurance.

CHIP is up for reauthorization in 2015

As of December 2013, 6 million children were covered under CHIP.

9.1 million children are enrolled or eligible to enroll in CHIP

2.7 million children need CHIP funding

6.4 million children would have access to other affordable health insurance coverage

1.6 million in CHIP fall into family glitch

645K uninsured fall into the family glitch

460K covered by CHIP funded Medicaid Expansion

1.3 million have affordable employer-sponsored family coverage

5.1 million eligible for Premium Tax Credits

AMERICAN ACTION
FORUM

As displayed in the chart above, the CHIP population has become fragmented, potentially leaving some children without coverage while others could join their families in Exchange or employer sponsored plans, and leaving some children without any coverage options, despite recent health care reform.

Features to Preserve in CHIP

CHIP was established as a product of bipartisan commitment, and any solution for the program should redirect the program on this path. Over the next few years, Congress will need an example of successful federal program reform with a responsible budgetary approach. For example, the Social Security Disability Insurance Trust Fund will become insolvent in 2016, and funding must be addressed. Congress should use CHIP funding to set the stage for productive, bipartisan solutions.

Along with setting an example for 2015 and 2016 legislative negotiations, this is an opportunity to utilize the successful design of CHIP to refine the population it set out to cover. In the time since its establishment, CHIP has become a swollen program, expanding beyond its original purpose. The changes to the program brought on by the ACA provide a unique opportunity to reassess who needs the program and who may not now that they have other options. Providing the appropriate amount of funding that is directed toward a specific population will preserve the program and its initial intentions for coverage.

One of the virtues of CHIP is that it is a state managed program; within the bounds of limited federal resources, Governors have the ability to design their programs in ways that best fit their state. This could be an extremely useful tool in redesigning the program, gaining insight into the best way to manage funding streams and address populations that may still need coverage in each state. It is important throughout this process to get the funding right for the future CHIP program. CHIP should be redesigned to meet the needs of a post-ACA health care system, while continuing the state determined personal responsibility provisions. Since states are the administrators of the program, any discussions of reauthorization should focus on allowing states to be more innovative and efficient in their ability to charge premiums, copays and enrollment fees. If these policy levers stay in place, states can tailor programs in a way that is beneficial for the program and allows the enrollee and their families to have greater involvement in their health care services.

Conclusion

This is only the first of what will be many discussions regarding options for the future of the CHIP program. This program was originally created in a bipartisan fashion, and any extension of the program should be approached in a bipartisan manner as well. CHIP provides millions of children with health insurance coverage. However, the ACA has changed the health care landscape and the types of coverage available to families, and the CHIP program must change as well.

Subsidized insurance is now available to many families currently enrolled in CHIP, and redundancies in coverage should be considered when making funding decisions, as should the children that are slipping through cracks in coverage created by the ACA. The $10 billion spent on this program in 2014 should not be taken as a given in years to come, and funding should be commensurate with the population needing coverage. CHIP coverage and funding must be assessed in the context of a changed health care landscape.

---

[1] Journal of Health and Social Policy. *The Impact of Lack of Health Insurance on Children.* *http://www.tandfonline.com/doi/abs/10.1300/J045v10n02_05#.VAnF0_mwIqc.*

[2] http://www.medicaid.gov/Medicaid-CHIP-Program-Information/By-Topics/Financing-and-Reimbursement/Childrens-Health-Insurance-Program-Financing.html

[3] http://kff.org/report-section/medicaid-enrollment-snapshot-december-2013-tables/

[4] http://www.kaiserhealthnews.org/stories/2014/may/21/aca-and-the-childrens-health-insurance-program.aspx

[5] http://ccf.georgetown.edu/chip/about-chip/

[6] This number includes the Medicaid program for the District of Columbia.

[7] http://www.medicaid.gov/Medicaid-CHIP-Program-Information/By-Topics/Childrens-Health-Insurance-Program-CHIP/Downloads/CHIPMap-01-14-13.pdf

[8] http://ccf.georgetown.edu/chip/about-chip/

[9] http://www.cbo.gov/sites/default/files/cbofiles/attachments/45653-OutlookUpdate_2014_Aug.pdf

[10] http://www.allhealth.org/briefingmaterials/RSAHRCHIP-FINAL[COLOR]_2L.PDF

[11] http://kff.org/report-section/medicaid-enrollment-snapshot-december-2013-tables/

[12] http://kff.org/report-section/medicaid-enrollment-snapshot-december-2013-tables/

[13] http://www.gao.gov/products/GAO-12-648

[14] http://americanactionforum.org/weekly-checkup/who-still-needs-chip

[15] http://americanactionforum.org/insights/chip-extension-and-how-the-aca-fails-families

[16] http://americanactionforum.org/weekly-checkup/who-still-needs-chip

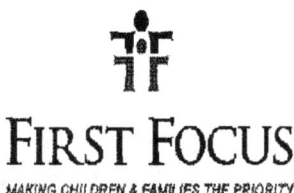

FIRST FOCUS

MAKING CHILDREN & FAMILIES THE PRIORITY

Testimony

Bruce Lesley

President, First Focus

Washington, D.C.

Senate Finance Committee
Subcommittee on Health Care

Hearing on

"The Children's Health Insurance Program:
Protecting America's Children and Families"

September 16, 2014

Thank you Chairman Rockefeller, Ranking Member Roberts, and members of the Finance Committee's Health Subcommittee for inviting me to speak to you today about the Children's Health Insurance Program (CHIP) and the positive impact it has had on the lives of millions of children across this country.

I would like to start by recognizing Chairman Rockefeller for his lifetime achievements in championing an array of issues, including child health, foster care, Supplemental Security Income (SSI), and child poverty, that have been critically important to the children of West Virginia and this entire country. As a former Senate staffer who worked for Senators Graham, Breaux, and Bingaman for over a decade, I witnessed Senator Rockefeller's passion and commitment to these issues up close and would like to personally thank him for his leadership on behalf of children, including his bipartisan work in this Committee with Senators Hatch, Kennedy, Chafee, and Grassley in helping create the Children's Health Insurance Program.

Mr. Chairman, CHIP has been an undeniable, bipartisan success story. As those of us that worked on the issue back in 1997 can attest, the lack of health insurance coverage among children was a national tragedy.

In fact, one in seven of our nation's children had no health insurance coverage and, in places like El Paso, Texas, where I grew up, the Public Health Department reported that nearly 40 percent of the children were living without health coverage and that families were just an illness away from tragedy or bankruptcy. I grew up with kids whose parents would not let them play sports out of fear that they would become injured and had a childhood classmate and friend who died tragically because his parents could not afford the expensive cancer treatment he needed to survive.

These were not isolated incidents. An Institute of Medicine (IOM) committee, which began analyzing the problems with children's health in 1996, found that "insurance coverage is the major determinant of whether children have access to health care" and that uninsured children are "most likely to be sick as newborns, less likely to be immunized as preschoolers, less likely to receive medical treatment when they are injured, and less likely to receive treatment for illnesses such as acute or recurrent ear infections, asthma, and tooth decay."

The report concluded:

> *Access to health care can influence children's physical and emotional growth, development, and overall health and well-being. Untreated illnesses and injuries can have long-term – even lifelong – consequences.*

And, according to a 1991 landmark report entitled *Beyond Rhetoric: A New American Agenda for Children and Families* by the bipartisan National Commission on Children, which was chaired by Senator Rockefeller:

Perhaps no set of issues moved members of the National Commission on Children more than the wrenching consequences of poor health and limited access to medical care. In urban centers and rural counties, we saw young children with avoidable illnesses and injuries, pregnant women without access to prenatal care, families whose emotional and financial resources were exhausted from providing special care for children with chronic illnesses and disabilities, and burned-out health care providers asked to do more than is humanly possible.

If this nation is to succeed in protecting children's health, there must be a major commitment from families, communities, health care providers, employers, and government to meet children's basic health needs and to ensure that all pregnant women and children have access to health care.

CHIP Is a National Success Story

Mr. Chairman, that commitment to protecting the health of our nation's children was answered by Congress in a bipartisan manner, with the passage of CHIP in 1997.

Through the leadership of Chairman Rockefeller and Senators Hatch, Kennedy, Chafee, Roth, and Moynihan in the Senate, the creation of CHIP was the result of a year-long debate and series of compromises that led to the commitment of $24 billion over seven years toward the goal of dramatically cutting the number of uninsured children in America.

The bipartisan discussions that senators had over the course of that year were inspiring. Although there were some disagreements about how the program should operate and compromises had to be found, the fact is that all of the members of the Finance Committee believed that we should no longer tolerate a situation where children should be sick, live in pain, or go without preventive care like vaccinations and annual check-ups just because their parents have lost their job or simply can't afford health insurance.

Democrats and Republicans agreed that investing in the health of our children is investing in America and its future. They recognized that when our children develop and thrive, we are paving the way for our country's next generation of workers and leaders. And when our kids aren't healthy, they do not learn and our nation will fail to stay the world's leader in innovation. That is why CHIP has proven to be so important.

Toward these goals, CHIP has been a rousing success story, as the uninsured rate for our nation's children has been cut in half – from 14 percent in 1997 to just 7 percent in 2012 (see Figure 1 from Kaiser Family Foundation) while the uninsured rate for adults (ages 18-64) has increased.

Figure 1

Uninsured Rates Among Nonelderly Adults and Children, 1997-2012

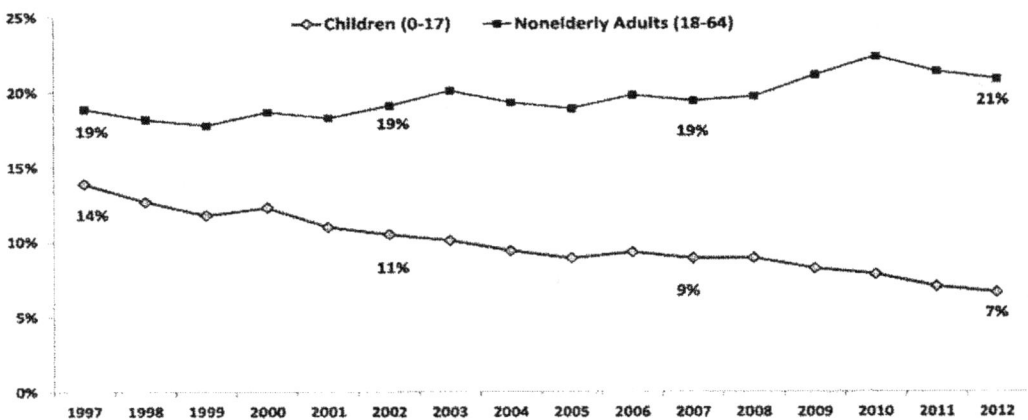

NOTE: Children includes all individuals under age 18.
SOURCE: KCMU analysis of the National Health Interview Survey data.

This past year, according to the Kaiser Family Foundation and the Congressional Budget Office (CBO), CHIP covered an average of 5.7 million children during a given month and over 8 million children for the year.

These success points exceed the expectations of many at the time CHIP was passed. For example, days before CHIP was passed by the U.S. Senate in 1997, Bobby Jindal, Louisiana's Director of Health and Hospitals (DHH) told Senator Breaux, whom I worked for at the time, that he thought it was highly unlikely that Louisiana would take up an expansion of coverage for children via CHIP.

However, although Louisiana was slow to act, the State did enact a program that was named LaCHIP. Louisiana's proposal to expand coverage to children was the 43rd plan approved by the federal government and, after a gradual phase-in of coverage over a couple of years, the State's program has proven to be incredibly successful. In fact, the uninsured rate for children in the Pelican State has, according to the U.S. Census Bureau, dropped from 23.2 percent in 1999 when LaCHIP was truly getting off the ground under Republican Governor Mike Foster and Democratic Governor Kathleen Blanco to 8.3 percent today under now Republican Governor Jindal.

Louisiana's positive experience is similar to that of most states across the country, as both Democratic and Republican governors and legislators have embraced and improved CHIP over the years so that today we are closing in on the bipartisan

National Commission on Children's goal and your vision, Senator Rockefeller, of ensuring that our nation's children and pregnant women have access to health care.

CHIP is also a program that has been tailored to the specific needs of children and pregnant women in the individual states. Recognizing that wages and health care costs are far different across the states, CHIP gives states discretion in working with their providers and insurance plans to set premiums, cost sharing, benefits, income eligibility levels, and provider networks for children and pregnant women rather than having a one-size-fits-all federal standard.

The downside to state flexibility has been that progress has been somewhat uneven. In 43 states and the District of Columbia, the uninsured rates for children are now below 12 percent and the rate is below 5 percent in the states of Massachusetts, Connecticut, Hawaii, Michigan, and Vermont.

In contrast, the rates of uninsured children, although much improved, tend to remain highest in the Southwest, where I grew up, and the South. Only seven states still have uninsured rates for children than exceed 12 percent and they are: Nevada, Texas, Alaska, Arizona (which is the only state in the country that has frozen CHIP), Florida, New Mexico, and Georgia (see Figure 2 from the Kaiser Family Foundation).

Figure 2

Uninsured Rates for Children by State, 2011-2012

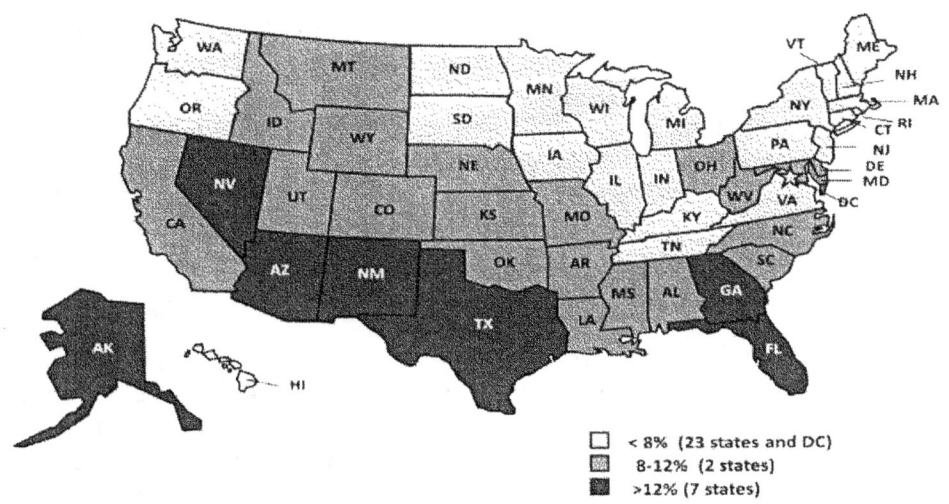

□ < 8% (23 states and DC)
▨ 8-12% (2 states)
■ >12% (7 states)

SOURCE: KCMU/Urban Institute analysis of the 2013 ASEC Supplement to the CPS.

Fortunately, we continue to make progress in closing in on the "finish line" of covering all kids. According to a report by Eugene Lewit at the Stanford University Center for Health Policy and Primary Care and Outcomes Research:

> *Approximately 88 percent of Medicaid or CHIP eligible children were enrolled in the programs in 2012. That was the highest rate of program participation for children among a number of other means-tested programs. It also represented an impressive increase in children's participation since the early years of CHIP and an increase of over six percentage points since just before the enactment of the Children's Health Insurance Program Reauthorization Act (CHIPRA) in February 2009.*

Nonetheless, an estimated 5 million of the remaining 7 million uninsured children in the country are eligible for but not enrolled in Medicaid and CHIP. Lewit found that groups with participation rates believe the national average include teenagers, children not living with their parents, Hispanic children, American Indian/Alaskan Native children, citizen children with noncitizen parent(s), eligible noncitizen children, and children with at least one parent eligible for Medicaid but unenrolled.

One of the hallmarks of CHIP has been the willingness of leaders on both sides of the aisle to work together to improve the enrollment of these children. For example, President George W. Bush championed a proposal to target eligible but unenrolled kids through outreach and enrollment grants. This initiative was incorporated into bipartisan legislation by Republican Majority Leader Frist and Senator Bingaman and was eventually included in CHIPRA. These grants have supported a number of community efforts to enroll into coverage some of our nation's most vulnerable children and have successfully helped drive down the uninsured rate of children.

Furthermore, Express Lane Enrollment is a streamlined process that facilitates Medicaid or CHIP enrollment for children based on verified eligibility criteria from other public assistance programs. This state option has been successfully adopted in a number of states, including Alabama, Colorado, Georgia, Iowa, Louisiana, Maryland, Maine, New Jersey, New York, Oklahoma, Pennsylvania, South Carolina, and Utah.

According to an evaluation of the program by Mathematica that was published this past December, the Express Lane Eligibility state option has been proven to reduce bureaucratic red tape and administrative costs while improving coverage rates in a number of states. Unfortunately, Express Lane Eligibility is currently slated to expire in March 2015. Instead, the state option should be extended permanently.

CHIP Is, by Definition, Child-Focused

CHIP is, as you know and by definition, child-focused and that has been a critical factor in its success for children. If you have talked to pediatricians or been inside a children's hospital, within the first five minutes, you have likely heard the mantra that "children are not little adults." As the IOM committee that issued the report entitled *America's Children: Health Insurance and Access to Care* in 1998 understood, children are better off if they are seen within a network of providers that have pediatric expertise and experience. The report recommended, "Public and private insurance should be encouraged to develop affordable products that address the specific needs of children, including children with chronic conditions and special health care needs."

Mr. Chairman and members of the Finance Committee, that is exactly what CHIP is. CHIP provider networks have been built and improved over the years in every single state and they must meet specific pediatric quality standards that address the unique developmental and health care needs of children.

According to the Assistant Secretary for Planning and Evaluation (ASPE) at the Department of Health and Human Services (HHS), "A survey of parents of CHIP enrollees in 10 states found that most CHIP enrollees (88 percent) had a usual source of care in the last 12 months and that 83 percent of CHIP parents found it usually or always easy to get appointments. The same survey also found that four-fifths of children received a preventive visit and 86 percent had a doctor or other health professional visit in 2012."

Similarly, a 2012 CHIP evaluation report by Mathematica Policy Research found, 92 percent of parents of CHIP enrollees never or rarely had problems paying their child's medical care. In sharp contrast, nearly half of the uninsured are not confident they can afford to pay for the health care services they need.

Therefore, CHIP has successfully expanded health coverage to kids, tailored services and benefits to address the special health care needs of children, improved access to health care, and reduced financial burdens for low-income families. In the face of a raft of bad news for children, including the fact that 22 percent of our America's kids are living in poverty, CHIP stands out as a shining success story.

In contrast, while the health of children and pregnant women are the first and only thought in CHIP, they can be an afterthought in the adult health care system, including private employer plans, the Federal Employees Health Benefits Program (FEHBP), and Marketplace exchange plans.

When I worked on Capitol Hill for Senator Bingaman, staff were shocked to hear at a briefing by FEHBP that program administrators did not even know how many children were served in the program and how some of the plans had very limited pediatric networks. One plan only listed a few pediatricians in all of Prince George's County, Maryland in its network and calls by staff found that even these few pediatricians were not accepting new patients. If you enrolled in that plan, lived in Prince George's County, and had kids, you would have been hard-pressed to find a primary care doctor for your child.

Worse, during one enrollment cycle, D.C.'s Children's Hospital was excluded from FEHBP's most popular Blue Cross plan option and it sent shock waves throughout the federal government as parents lined up at Office of Personnel Management (OPM) enrollment booths to get information on how to change their insurance option to protect their children's access to care. Unfortunately, when parents changed their plans, it was often at the expense of losing their own provider networks, and I can personally attest that this was a disaster for many of us.

Subsequently, with the advent of the insurance exchanges in the Affordable Care Act (ACA), although we strongly support important provisions related to bans on pre-existing condition exclusions or lifetime caps that were so harmful to a number of children, there remains a number of issues that need to be worked out for kids. For example, just this past week, Seattle Children's Hospital resolved a lawsuit and lengthy negotiation with insurers, including Premera Blue Cross and Regence in Washington State, to ensure that the Children's Hospital can be included as an available provider option to children in the State's exchange plans.

CHIP Plays a Key Role in Reducing Health Disparities

CHIP, in partnership with Medicaid, serves as an important source of coverage for children of all races and ethnicities. According to the Kaiser Family Foundation, about a quarter of white (26 percent) and Asian-American (25 percent) children, and over half of African-American (54 percent) and Hispanic (52 percent) children are served by Medicaid and CHIP.

According to the HHS Action Plan to Reduce Racial and Ethnic Health Disparities, one of the foremost action strategies of the Secretary is to "increase the proportion of people with health insurance and provide patient protections in Medicaid, CHIP, Medicare, health insurance exchanges, and other forms of health insurance."

As noted earlier, strategies that include outreach and enrollment grants and the use of Express Lane Eligibility are important mechanisms to reduce the number of uninsured and disparities in health coverage.

One example of this is to better utilize community health workers or "promotoras" to help uninsured but eligible children get enrolled into coverage but to also assist families in navigating the health care system to ensure their children receive the insurance benefits and public health services that their kids need.

"Such activities will have a focus on reducing disparities in coverage for racial and ethnic minorities and those experiencing language barriers," according to the Action Plan. "Linking enrollment of children and families in CHIP and Medicaid to enrollment in human service programs will improve the access and availability of both health care and human services for underserved populations."

Therefore, in addition to extending CHIP's funding, it is important that Congress also extend the authorization and funding for both outreach and enrollment efforts that include the use of community health workers or "promotoras" and Express Lane Eligibility.

And, beyond coverage improvements, a study published by the National Institutes of Health (NIH) found that CHIP coverage has been critically important and successful in reducing disparities in access to care measures, including usual source of care (USC), preventive care use, unmet needs, patterns of USC use, and parent-rated quality of care between white children and black or Hispanic children. However, more work needs to be done in terms of addressing language barriers, improving provider workforce diversity, and expanding quality initiatives to drive further reductions in health disparities.

Rural Children Would Stand to Lose the Most if CHIP Expires

As a former Senate staffer to the Senate Rural Health Caucus, I know that many of you are deeply concerned about the impact that health policy has in rural communities. Consequently, First Focus commissioned a study of the uninsured rate and coverage rates of Medicaid and CHIP in both rural and urban communities and found what may be a surprising result to some.

In this study by William O'Hare entitled *Rural Children Increasingly Rely on Medicaid and State Child Health Insurance Programs for Health Insurance*, he analyzed Census Bureau data for child health coverage and his key findings include:

- *The percent of children who lack health insurance is the same in both urban and rural areas but the source of insurance coverage differs.*
- *Of the fifty counties with the highest rate of uninsured children, 45 are rural counties.*
- *In 2012, 52 percent of rural children lived in low-income families (those with income less than 200 percent of the poverty line) compared to 42 percent of urban children.*
- *Children in rural areas are more reliant on health insurance from public sources. In 2012, 47 percent of rural children are covered by public insurance compared to 38 percent of urban children.*

Due to the higher levels of child poverty in rural America, where over half the children live in families with income below 200 percent of the poverty line, the uninsured rate for children would be much higher if it were not for the health coverage offered by Medicaid and CHIP.

In fact, if CHIP were to be allowed to expire, it is clear the result would be negative to both rural and urban children, but that the children in rural America would stand the most to lose and would be disproportionately harmed.

Even worse, for those rural communities that already have some of the highest uninsured rates for children in the country, the loss of CHIP would compound what is already an enormous problem.

CHIP is Overwhelmingly Popular with the American People

In light of the importance that CHIP plays in the lives of millions of children and the many successes that CHIP has had since its inception 17 years ago, it is not surprising that the American people know a good thing when they see it.

In November 2008, a Lake Research Partners survey found that American voters supported renewing CHIP, which was facing expiration in March 2009, by a resounding 82-10 percent margin.

Four years later, another Election Eve poll by Lake Research Partners found that, despite the partisanship and acrimony that had developed around the Affordable Care Act (ACA), voters in both political parties overwhelmingly supported extending CHIP by a wide 83-13 percent margin.

And in May of this year, a poll by American Viewpoint found that voters continue to support extending CHIP by a margin of 74-14 percent.

At a time when one-quarter of the American people seem to be so disenchanted and cynical that they oppose just about everything, it is a testament to CHIP that it has maintained such strong bipartisan support over the years. The same is true when the pool breaks down support by age, gender, and racial groups.

In the American Viewpoint poll, for example, the level of support versus opposition to extending CHIP is:

- 80-10 percent among Democrats
- 66-19 percent among Republicans
- 75-15 percent among Independents
- 66-18 percent among self-identified "Tea Party supporters"
- 77-12 percent among women
- 71-16 percent among men
- 80-9 percent among adults 18-29 years of age
- 72-15 percent among adults over the age of 65
- 72-14 percent among whites
- 79-14 percent among African-Americans
- 79-12 percent among Hispanics
- 79-13 percent among parents
- 73-16 percent among grandparents
- 71-15 percent among adults without children

- 76-14 percent among urban voters
- 74-15 percent among suburban voters
- 72-13 percent among rural voters
- 75-15 percent in states where both senators are Republicans
- 71-13 percent in states where the senators are split
- 76-14 percent in states where both senators are Democrats

No matter how you break it down, American voters support CHIP by wide margins.

Unfortunately, CHIP's 8 Million Children Are at Risk

Although CHIP celebrated its 17th birthday this year and has achieved a remarkable record of success, funding for the program expires on September 30, 2015, and there is some urgency to addressing the issue as soon as possible because states are beginning their budget preparation now and are facing uncertainly about how to handle CHIP beginning in October 2015. In addition to the state's budget planning needs, states also need to resign contracts with private health plans and those private health plans need to resign contracts with their health care providers for the upcoming year.

Unfortunately, with the establishment of the ACA Marketplace plans, there are some that are questioning whether CHIP should be extended after September 2015. The problem is that, if CHIP funding were allowed to expire – either purposely or due to congressional inaction – it is estimated that up to 2 million children who currently rely on CHIP's coverage for their asthma, vision, dental, or cancer treatment would become uninsured unless they are able to obtain alternative coverage through some alternative source, such as Medicaid, the exchange plans, employer coverage, or the individual market.

In analyzing the question of what would happen to the health coverage of 8 million children if CHIP were allowed to expire, the Medicaid and CHIP Payment and Access Commission (MACPAC) issued a report in June which "found that many children now served by the program would not have a smooth transition to another source of coverage" and that the "number of uninsured children would likely rise...."

One of the major factors, according to researchers at the Urban Institute, is that "as many as half of the children with Medicaid or CHIP coverage and family incomes above 138 percent of poverty might not qualify for Marketplace subsidies if CHIP were not reauthorized." This is because the ACA precludes families from receiving exchange subsidies to purchase coverage if they are made an offer of "affordable" employer-sponsored coverage to an individual employee, even if the cost of health coverage for the entire family is "unaffordable." This problem is referred to as either the "family glitch" or "kid glitch" in the ACA.

But, even for those that would be able to make the leap from CHIP to the qualified health plans (QHPs) in the Marketplaces, the Wakely Consulting Group, on behalf of the Robert Wood Johnson Foundation, compared the actuarial value and benefits offered by CHIP plans to QHPs in 35 states.

In their report entitled *Comparison of Benefits and Cost Sharing in Children's Health Insurance Programs to Qualified Health Plans*, the Wakely Group found that children are currently offered excellent and superior pediatric-focused coverage through CHIP than they could obtain through the Marketplaces (see Figure 3).

Figure 3: Wakely Group Comparison of Cost Sharing and Benefits in CHIP versus Exchange Plans

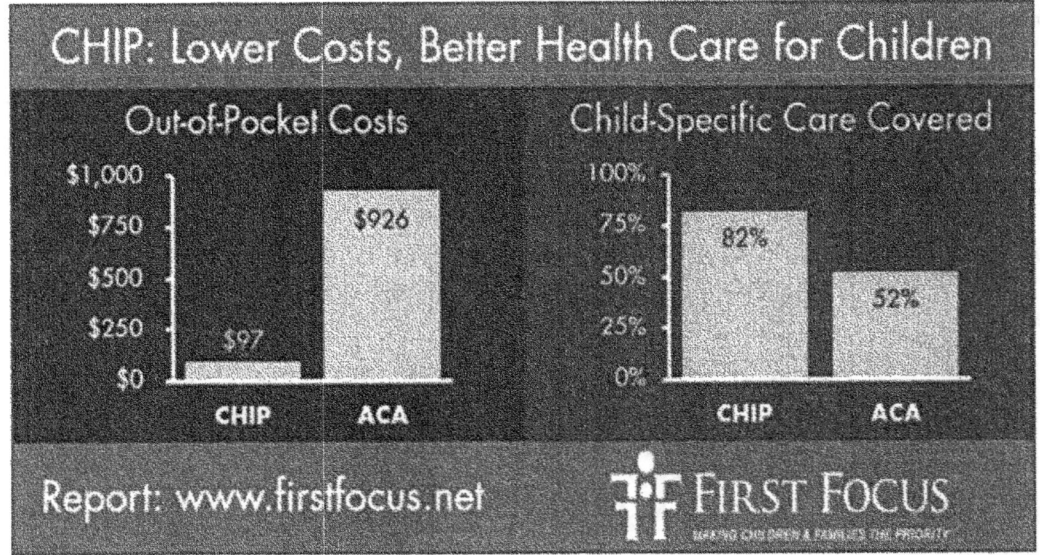

The report's findings include:

• **Average Cost Sharing**: In every state, children covered by CHIP would have significantly lower levels of cost sharing than through plans offered on the exchanges. For example, the Wakely Group found that the average cost sharing for a child in CHIP is estimated at $97 for households with incomes at 210 percent of the federal poverty level (FPL) compared to $926, which is 955 percent higher, for a child in the exchanges. In every single one of the 35 states studied, CHIP cost sharing is much lower than the level of cost sharing required in QHPs through the exchanges. **CHIP is superior**

• **Total Out-Of-Pocket Costs**: Children with special health care needs that are currently served by CHIP would be hardest hit by a transition to QHPs. In some states, children with special health care needs could go from paying $0 in cost sharing in CHIP to over $5,000 in annual out-of-pocket expenditures in the exchange plans. **CHIP is superior**

• **Coverage of Benefits and Services**: CHIP covers more child-specific services and benefits with fewer limits than QHPs. For example, CHIP covers more child-specific services and benefits, such as pediatric dental, vision, hearing, autism services, habilitation, etc., than QHPs in the exchanges.

As an example, on the issue of pediatric dental coverage, QHPs can exclude dental benefits if a stand-alone dental plan is available in that state. As a result, only 40 percent of QHPs that were reviewed offer pediatric dental as an embedded benefit in the QHP. In more than half of the states studied, children moving from CHIP plans into QHPs would likely need to purchase separate stand-alone dental plans in order to have comparable coverage, which means that families would face additional costs for the separate premium required in a stand-alone dental plan. **CHIP is superior**

• **Benefit Limits or Caps**: Even with respect to benefits that are provided through both CHIP and QHPs, the Wakely Group found that CHIP plans have fewer limits or caps that are imposed on that coverage.

For instance, with respect to physical, occupational, and speech therapy, the Wakely study found that both CHIP and QHPs cover all of these services. However, four-fifths, or 80 percent, of QHPs impose utilizations limits and caps for these services, which is in sharp contrast to 42 percent of CHIP plans. **CHIP is superior**

In all 35 states studied and analyzed by the Wakely Group, if children were transitioned from CHIP to exchange QHPs, they would face significantly higher out-of-pocket costs and have fewer child-specific benefits covered. In short, millions of children would be left worse off if Congress fails to extend CHIP.

• **Child-Centered Networks**: But, even beyond the lower cost-sharing and stronger benefits, CHIP is important to protect because the health provider networks in CHIP are made up largely with doctors, nurses, and hospitals that have pediatric and maternal child health expertise. They are educated and trained to recognize and treat the unique array of physical, mental, social, and emotional developmental needs of children as they grow from infancy through adolescence. This focused attention and expertise in addressing children's special needs stands in sharp contrast to the situation in other types of adult-centered coverage.

For example, while a CHIP quality review panel's time is spent almost entirely reviewing and discussing ways to improve child health, child advocates have found it difficult to even get even one pediatric expert to be named to such a panel in adult-centered networks or to get time focused on the needs of children.

According to analysis by the Urban Institute, just 1-2 percent of all spending in the health reform Marketplaces is projected to be attributable to children's coverage, so

attention to the cost and quality of care for kids will simply not be a top priority.
CHIP is superior

Conclusion and Recommendations

Toward the end of World War I, the United States Children's Bureau and Woman's Committee of the Council of National Defense issued a decree in April 1918 that declared: "The health of the child is the power of the nation." They recognized that the health of children is a cornerstone to ensuring both their and the nation's long-term well-being and success.

Over the years, our nation's leaders have chosen to make some key strategic investments toward these goals of improving the lives of children and securing our nation's long-term success. In 1997, even amidst a discussion to pass a major deficit reduction package, the Congress – beginning with leadership in this Committee – chose to make such an investment to improve the health of our nation's children.

This has proven to be a wise investment, as CHIP has – in partnership with Medicaid – cut the uninsured rate for our nation's children in half over its 17 years. Since its beginning, CHIP has been a bipartisan, state-administered, public-private partnership that has always understood that "children are not little adults" and have unique developmental needs that often require pediatric expertise.

CHIP has also made important strides in reducing health disparities. And, despite two recessions and the resulting increase in child poverty, CHIP and Medicaid have managed to keep reducing the uninsured rate of children while the uninsured rates for adults were heading in the other direction. Consequently, the American public recognizes its value and, by overwhelming margins, strongly support its continuation.

In short, CHIP works and works well.

Nevertheless, with the passage of the ACA, there are some that have questioned whether we or not we should fold CHIP into the Marketplace exchanges. However, when you look at all the evidence, research from the Wakely Consulting Group, the Urban Institute, MACPAC, the American Academy of Pediatrics, the National Academy for State Health Policy, the Georgetown Center for Children and Families, the Children's Dental Health Project, the March of Dimes, the National Alliance to Advance Adolescent Health, and First Focus all point to the fact that, although the ACA holds great promise for millions of uninsured adults who otherwise lack affordable coverage options, allowing CHIP to expire would leave millions of children without health coverage and millions of others worse off unless significant legislative and regulatory improvements are made to the ACA.

Much would need to be improved in the exchanges and the law before Congress should consider moving children from CHIP to the Marketplace plans or else millions of children would be left worse off.

Consequently, over 400 organizations representing all 50 states have signed a joint letter urging Congress to, as soon as possible, protect and fully extend CHIP into the future.

Recommendations

Specifically, we urge Congress to adopt a **four-year extension of CHIP funding** through 2019. This would rightfully align the funding with the program's reauthorization date and we urge the Congress to pass such an extension during the lame duck session, as there is some urgency to this.

In fact, although CHIP funding does not expire until September 30, 2015, states are beginning to put together their budgets for FY 2016 now and state agencies are working with managed care organizations and providers across the country on CHIP network contracts. They are looking to the Congress for some assurances that the program will continue as they do their work.

We would also urge the **extension of outreach and enrollment grants, the pediatric quality standards, and Express Lane Eligibility** (which expires in March 2015) so that we continue to make progress toward the goal of covering all children.

And, although it is a Medicaid issue, we would also like to express our support for legislation by Senators Murray and Brown entitled the "Ensuring Access to Primary Care for Women and Children Act," as it would provide a 2-year extension to a provision in the ACA that raised Medicaid payments for certain primary care services up to Medicare levels. This **extension of the pay parity provision** would help improve access to care for children and pregnant women in the Medicaid program but it is currently set to expire on Dec. 31, 2014.

In closing, I would like to once again thank Chairman Rockefeller and Ranking Member Roberts for holding this important hearing about children's health. This Committee has always provided the leadership on CHIP and we look forward to working with you all toward its extension.

I would also like to personally recognize and thank Chairman Rockefeller for his outstanding career as a champion for our nation's most vulnerable citizens: its children. We appreciate all that you have done over the years for kids. Thank you!

United States Senate Subcommittee on Health
Public Hearing
"The Children's Health Insurance Program: Protecting America's Children and Families"
September 16, 2014

Responses to Questions for the Record From Bruce Lesley

<u>**Senate Finance Committee Chairman Wyden:**</u>

The Children's Health Insurance Program works well for millions of children and families. The Affordable Care Act is also going to make a huge difference in the lives of Americans across the country. However, we are still working through some technical issues that have real impacts on families. On such example is the "kid glitch," which may leave millions of children without access to affordable coverage.

Question #1: Mr. Lesley, can you discuss the impact of the "kid glitch" on families and children and provide detail on how many children would be left without access to affordable coverage if funding for the Children's Health Insurance Program is not extended?

Answer: If the Children's Health Insurance Program was not extended by Congress, an estimated 2 million children would be denied coverage in the Marketplace because of what is referred to as the "kid glitch." This is because the ACA denies tax credits to those workers who are determined to have access to "affordable" employer coverage, and "affordability" is defined as an employee having an offer of coverage through their employer that would cost less than 9.5 percent of his or her income. The problem here is that "affordability" is based on the cost of individual coverage relative to a workers' wages rather than the cost of a family policy.

For example, in 2014, according to a Kaiser Family Foundation benefits study, the average premium contributions for private sector insurance coverage was $6,025 for single coverage and $16,834 for family coverage. As a result, premiums for family coverage are 2.8 times more expensive than that for individuals.

Even worse, although employers often help out with the cost of this coverage, they often provide reduced support for the added expense of family coverage. As a result, Kaiser Family Foundation estimates that the average employee pays $1,081 in premiums for single coverage and $4,823 for family coverage. Put another way, the family premium is 446 percent more expensive to the average employee than for the individual.

This is particularly problematic for children because the ACA's "affordability test" fails to take into account this wide disparity in costs between single and family coverage, and so dependents are disproportionately harmed by the provision's interpretation. Due to this impact on family or dependent coverage, the provision's interpretation has been referred to as either the "family glitch" or the "kid glitch."

Consequently, if CHIP were allowed to expire, an estimated 2 million children that are currently enrolled in CHIP would be left without access to Marketplace tax credits and become uninsured.

Health Subcommittee Chairman Rockefeller:

Question #1: CHIP COVERAGE FOR RURAL CHILDREN:

In my state of West Virginia, many people are both sicker and older than the rest of the American population. And this is true for many rural states across the country. Regardless of your age, in rural areas—which are also burdened with high levels of unemployment and poverty—it is often more difficult to access health care services because families live in remote areas.

Given these barriers, and the high levels of chronic disease in rural America, it is critically important that rural children have access to health insurance in order to receive the care they need for a fair shot in life.

Mr. Lesley, how would rural children, like those in West Virginia, be impacted should the CHIP program come to end as we know it?

Answer: According to a recent report we released, rural children in this country rely more heavily on getting their health coverage through either Medicaid or CHIP than urban children. Nationally, 47 of rural children and 38 percent of urban children are enrolled in either Medicaid or CHIP. Those are the exact same percentages of enrollment in West Virginia.

The higher percentage of rural children enrolled in Medicaid and CHIP than urban children is attributable to the fact that rural children are far more likely to live in households with income below 200 percent of the poverty level (52 percent compared to 42 percent for urban children).

Consequently, if CHIP were allowed to expire, rural children in both West Virginia and across the entire country would be disproportionately harmed and health disparities would increase.

Question #2: TRANSITIONS:

The last time Congress extended CHIP, we included a provision requiring careful study of the transition process for children to flesh out the benefits of CHIP versus other sources of coverage. This study is not due for eight months (April 2015) and I am growing concerned that there is minimal data and infrastructure to assist children in a transition from CHIP to other coverage at this time.

Mr. Lesley, could you describe the safeguards you would recommend, from a policy perspective, before children could responsibly be moved between plans?

Answer: For children, there are a number of important factors that are important to them for their health care coverage. The first among them is benefits. According to a recent report commissioned by the Robert Wood Johnson Foundation with the Wakely Consulting Group, CHIP provides a much stronger and wider array of benefits than the coverage offered by plans in the ACA Marketplace or the private sector. The most glaring example of this is the dental benefit, which is guaranteed as a benefit in CHIP but is rarely included in the ACA Marketplace plans or the private sector and often must be purchased separately. Furthermore, habilitative services for children with special health care needs and other child-specific benefits are much stronger in CHIP than in the ACA Marketplace or the private sector. In fact, CHIP plans are nearly twice as likely as Qualified Health Plans (QHPs) in the Marketplace to cover child-specific benefits with no limits.

For low-income working families, affordability is also critically important and CHIP is far superior for children than what is offered in either the ACA Marketplace or the private sector. In fact, according to the Wakely Consulting Group report, "The most significant impact for CHIP enrollees transitioning to QHPs was a substantial increase in estimated out of pocket costs at the point of care (deductibles, copays, and/or coinsurance)." For example, at 210 percent of poverty, the average annual cost sharing for a child enrolled in CHIP was estimated to be $97 compared to the average of $926, or 955 percent greater, for a child enrolled in a QHP.

In response to your previous question, I noted that the "kid glitch" would need to be corrected or an estimated 2 million children could lose coverage entirely. Assuring comparability would also require addressing this problem, although it is our understanding that the Office of Management and Budget has estimated that such a fix would require billions of dollars in new spending. Furthermore, children are not little adults and have special health care needs that often require pediatric expertise and knowledge. CHIP recognizes this fact and, as a result, states contract with managed care companies and providers that are, by definition, focused almost entirely on delivering pediatric and maternity care services. CHIP also has a number of pediatric quality measures that CHIP networks are accountable to meet.

In sharp contrast, children represent a very small fraction of the enrollees in the ACA Marketplace and, therefore, there is little focus on ensuring strong pediatrics networks and quality in the QHPs. In fact, according to the Urban Institute, spending on children in the ACA Marketplace is estimated to be only 1-2 percent of all costs, so children are almost an afterthought. As a result, CHIP networks are far more robust and critically important pediatric providers have been left out entirely by some QHPs, which are almost entirely focused on adults.

Therefore, if Congress were to choose to move kids from CHIP to the ACA Marketplace and wanted to ensure that no child would be left worse off, Congress and the Administration would have to enact legislation that would include a number of safeguards, including provisions to strengthen the benefits, reduce the cost sharing, eliminate the "kid glitch," expand pediatric networks, and implement pediatric-specific quality standards within the ACA Marketplace. Such legislation would be extremely complex because CHIP eligibility, benefits, and cost sharing differs from state to state and federal legislation would have a nearly impossible time of addressing such variation. Such legislation would also be expensive because CHIP currently delivers stronger benefits and lower cost sharing to its enrollees at a lower average cost than QHPs.

Senator Cantwell:

Mr. Lesley, I am concerned that if federal funding were to expire for CHIP at the end of fiscal year 2015, the vast majority of CHIP-covered children in Washington (more than 45,000) would be forced to find coverage through Qualified Health Plans. Given that many low-income adults who currently have coverage through Qualified Health Plans are struggling to afford their premiums and cost-sharing responsibilities, I am concerned that switching children to exchange plans may make their health coverage inaccessible or cost-prohibitive.

Question #1: Do you have any evidence of the comparability between the cost-sharing for a typical beneficiary in CHIP versus the cost-sharing for a typical beneficiary on a state or federally-run exchange?

Answer: You are correct. Affordability within CHIP is far superior for children than what is offered in either the ACA Marketplace or the private sector. According to the Wakely Consulting Group report, "The most significant impact for CHIP enrollees transitioning to QHPs was a substantial increase in estimated out of pocket costs at the point of care (deductibles, copays, and/or coinsurance)." For example, at 210 percent of poverty, the average annual cost sharing for a child enrolled in CHIP was estimated to be $97 compared to the average of $926, or 955 percent greater, for a child enrolled in a QHP.

Question #2: Do you have any evidence on what the difference would be in Washington State?

Answer: The wide disparity at the national level is even greater in Washington State. In fact, a child enrolled in Washington's CHIP program at 210 percent of poverty has no out of pocket costs, while the average annual cost sharing in the QHPs is estimated to be between $891–$960 a year. And, for a child with special health care needs, CHIP imposes no cost sharing on children while the family would have to spend $5,200 to reach their out of pocket maximum in a QHP. For working families with children at that income level, such an added expense could be devastating.

Question #3: If coverage is disrupted for these children, is it possible that any of these children would become uninsured, and if so, how would that impact the health of these children and the continuity of their health care?

Answer: If CHIP was not extended by Congress, an estimated 2 million children would become uninsured because they would be unable to transition to coverage in the Marketplace because of what is referred to as the "kid glitch." They clearly would be left much worse off.

It is important to note that there are some children that would be able to meet the "affordability test" and quality for tax credits in the ACA Marketplace, but they would also be left worse off. According to an analysis by the Wakely Consulting Group for the Robert Wood Johnson Foundation, they determined that children would find fewer benefits, more limits on benefits, and have much greater cost sharing in the ACA Marketplace plans than they currently receive in CHIP.

Moreover, as has been the case in Washington State, we have seen a number of instances where pediatric provider networks are much weaker in the ACA Marketplace plans than in CHIP. For example, a number of the QHPs failed to include Seattle Children's Hospital in their provider networks. Although bad publicity and a lawsuit inspired the plans to adjust their networks to include Seattle Children's Hospital, we are hearing lots of stories where children are having a difficult time finding access to pediatric specialty care services in QHPs, as those networks are narrower in terms of pediatrics than what is offered in CHIP. For families that rely on a certain children's hospital or a pediatric specialist to take care of their child's health care needs, this could be devastating to their treatment plan and their continuity of care.

As you may know, Section 2105(g) of the Social Security Act allows Washington to use CHIP funds to pay the difference between the Medicaid Federal Medical Assistance Program (FMAP) match rate and the enhanced CHIP matching rate for Medicaid-financed children whose family income exceeds 133 percent of the federal poverty level.

Question #4: What would the impact be in states such as mine if Section 2105(g) is altered or discontinued in a future CHIP reauthorization?

Answer: Section 2105(g) was an important provision added to CHIP to improve fairness in the allocation of funding to the states, as CHIP initially penalized states in their allotments if they had expanded coverage to children above the minimal levels required in Medicaid prior to the enactment of CHIP. For states such as Washington, they were effectively penalized for being leaders on covering children.

Section 2105(g) addressed this inequity. If it were altered in a negative fashion or discontinued in a future CHIP reauthorization, this would restore the inequity and penalty to those states that had forged the pathway toward expanding health coverage to children upon which CHIP followed.

The New York Times

SUNDAYREVIEW   NYT NOW

The Way to Beat Poverty

By NICHOLAS KRISTOF and SHERYL WuDUNN   SEPT. 12, 2014

AS our children were growing up, one of their playmates was a girl named Jessica. Our kids would disappear with Jessica to make forts, build a treehouse and share dreams. We were always concerned because — there's no polite way to say this — Jessica was a mess.

Her mother, a teen mom, was away in prison for drug-related offenses, and Jessica had never known her father. While Jessica was very smart, she used her intelligence to become a fluent, prodigious liar. Even as a young girl, she seemed headed for jail or pregnancy, and in sixth grade she was kicked out of school for bringing alcohol to class. One neighbor forbade his daughter to play with her, and after she started setting fires we wondered if we should do the same.

Jessica reminded us that the greatest inequality in America is not in wealth but the even greater gap of opportunity. We had been trying to help people in Zimbabwe and Cambodia, and now we found ourselves helpless to assist one of our daughter's best friends.

One reason the United States has not made more progress against poverty is that our interventions come too late. If there's one overarching lesson from the past few decades of research about how to break the cycles of poverty in the United States, it's the power of parenting — and of intervening early, ideally in the first year or two of life or even before a child is born.

Within four weeks of conception, a human embryo has formed a neural tube, which then begins to produce brain cells. As the brain is forming, it is shaped by the uterine environment in ways that will affect the child for the rest of his or her life. A mother who drinks alcohol may leave her child with fetal alcohol syndrome or, less serious, fetal alcohol effects. A study by Ann Streissguth at the University of Washington found that by age 14, 60 percent of children born with fetal alcohol syndrome or effects have been suspended from school or expelled. Almost half have displayed inappropriate sexual behavior such as public masturbation.

Children with fetal alcohol effects account for 1 percent of births; 20 percent of births in America are to mothers who smoked during pregnancy. These babies have smaller head circumferences on average, and because nicotine increases the testosterone in the woman's uterus, some theorize that this may lead to a greater penchant for aggressiveness, particularly among sons. Patricia A. Brennan of Emory University found that when a mother smoked a pack a day during pregnancy, her offspring were more than twice as likely to be violent criminals as adults.

Likewise, when a pregnant woman is exposed to lead from old paint or from air pollution, her fetus absorbs it in ways that impair the development of the brain. Some research suggests that the rise of crime in the mid-20th century may have been caused in part by the increasing presence of lead in the environment, and that one factor in the decline in crime from the 1990s on was the phasing out of lead from gasoline (and thus from air pollution) beginning two decades earlier.

The lifelong impact of what happens early in life was reinforced by a series of studies on laboratory rats by Michael Meaney of McGill University in Canada. Professor Meaney noticed that some rat mothers were always licking and grooming their pups (baby rats are called pups), while others were much less attentive. He found that rats that had been licked and cuddled as pups were far more self-confident, curious and intelligent. They were also better at mazes, healthier and longer-lived.

Professor Meaney mixed up the rat pups, taking biological offspring of the licking mothers and giving them at birth to the moms who licked less. Then he took pups born to the laissez-faire mothers and gave them to be raised by those committed to licking and grooming. When the pups grew up, he ran them through the same battery of tests. What mattered, it turned out, wasn't biological parentage but whether a rat pup was licked and groomed attentively.

The licking and grooming seemed to affect the development of brain structures that regulate stress. A rat's early life in a lab is highly stressful (especially when scientists are picking up the pups and handling them), leading to the release of stress hormones such as cortisol. In the rats with less attentive mothers, the cortisol shaped their brains to prepare for a life of danger and stress. But the attentive mothers used their maternal licking and grooming to soothe their pups immediately, dispersing the cortisol and leaving their brains unaffected.

A series of studies have found similar patterns in humans. Scientists can measure cortisol in an infant's saliva, and babies turn out to be easily stressed. Anything from loud noises to hunger to a soiled diaper floods the child's brain with cortisol. But when Mom or Dad hugs the child, the stress and cortisol almost disappear. If a baby is in a bassinet and gets a shot, its cortisol level soars; if the mom is holding the baby, the cortisol level rises, but much more modestly.

Dr. Jack P. Shonkoff, founder of the Center on the Developing Child at Harvard University, has been a pioneer in this research. He argues that the constant bath of cortisol in a high-stress infancy prepares the child for a high-risk environment. The cortisol affects brain structures so that those individuals are on a fight-or-flight hair trigger throughout life, an adaptation that might have been useful in prehistory. But in today's world, the result is schoolchildren who are so alert to danger that they cannot concentrate. They are also so suspicious of others that they are prone to pre-emptive aggression.

Dr. Shonkoff calls this "toxic stress" and describes it as one way that poverty regenerates. Moms in poverty often live in stressful homes while juggling a thousand challenges, and they are disproportionately likely to be teenagers, without a partner to help out. A baby in such an environment is more likely to grow up with a brain bathed in cortisol.

Fortunately, a scholar named David Olds has shown that there are ways to snap this poverty cycle.

Mr. Olds began his career working with 4-year-olds, but then decided that many children were already traumatized and damaged at that age, so he needed to start earlier. He founded an initiative that became Nurse-Family Partnership, dispatching nurses to visit low-income, disadvantaged families and offer counseling on child-rearing. The nurses begin visiting during pregnancy, urging moms not to drink or use drugs while carrying a baby.

One nurse, Stacy, worked with a pregnant 17-year-old named Bonnie, who lived in a dirt-floor basement apartment. Bonnie smoked, drank, got into fistfights and regularly collided with the law. When Stacy suggested that Bonnie stop smoking, Bonnie threatened to slap her. "This baby's taken everything else away from me," Bonnie raged. "It's not going to take away my cigarettes."

It turned out that Bonnie had been abused as a child and had, as a babysitter, abused others as well. During one of Stacy's visits, she broke down and confessed her fear of abusing her own child — "especially if it's a crier." Stacy suggested some coping mechanisms and wrote down the name of an older woman living nearby whom Bonnie could call for help. Stacy taped the paper to the wall, ready for a crisis. Bonnie did call the older woman, who helped out, and against all odds Bonnie ended up taking quite good care of her baby — which may be why that child ended up graduating from high school many years later. These nurse visits continue until the child turns 2, with the nurse encouraging the mom to speak to the child constantly, to read to the child, to show affection. Later there are discussions of birth control.

The visits have been studied extensively through randomized controlled trials — the gold standard of evidence — and are stunningly effective. Children randomly assigned to nurse visits suffer 79 percent fewer cases of state-verified abuse or neglect than similar children randomly assigned to other programs. Even though the program ends at age 2, the children at age 15 have fewer than half as many arrests on average. At the 15-year follow-up, the mothers themselves have one-third fewer subsequent births and have spent 30 fewer months on welfare than the controls. A RAND Corporation study found that each dollar invested in nurse visits to low-income unmarried mothers produced $5.70 in benefits.

So here we have an anti-poverty program that is cheap, is backed by rigorous evidence and pays for itself several times over in reduced costs later on.

Yet it has funds to serve only 2 percent to 3 percent of needy families. That's infuriating.

There are a couple of lessons we can learn from David Olds and from other programs with a solid record of proven effectiveness. First, it is critical to intervene early, in the crucial window when the brain is developing and the foundations for adult life are being laid. That means helping women avert pregnancies they don't want and, if they become pregnant, helping them deflect dangers such as drug use, alcohol and tobacco.

James Heckman, a Nobel Prize-winning economist at the University of Chicago, says that our society would be better off taking sums we invest in high school and university and redeploying them to help struggling kids in the first five years of life. We certainly would prefer not to cut education budgets of any kind, but if pressed, we would have to agree that $1 billion spent on home visitation for at-risk young mothers would achieve much more in breaking the poverty cycle than the same sum spent on indirect subsidies collected by for-profit universities.

Second, children's programs are most successful when they leverage the most important — and difficult — job in the world: parenting. Give parents the tools to nurture their child in infancy and the result will be a more self-confident and resilient person for decades to come. It's far less expensive to coach parents to support children than to maintain prisons years later.

What does that mean for all of us? We wish more donors would endow not just professorships but also the jobs of nurses who visit at-risk parents; we wish tycoons would seek naming opportunities not only at concert halls and museum wings but also in nursery schools. We need advocates to push federal, state and local governments to invest in the first couple of years of life, to support parents during pregnancy and a child's earliest years.

As for our children's friend, Jessica, she's now 20. She was taken in by a wonderful foster family in high school and began to thrive. She became the first person in her family to go to college, but then the money ran out after freshman year, so she's working and planning to go back to school later. We think she'll pull it off — but her troubled journey underscores that it's always better to help young children at the front end, rather than try to undo the damage later.

If you want to help, here are a few organizations whose work on early childhood has impressed us.

NURSE-FAMILY PARTNERSHIP is a proven home-visitation program that gives at-risk kids a shot at reaching the starting line. *nursefamilypartnership.org*

REACH OUT AND READ supports pediatricians who hand out books to low-income children during doctor visits, with instructions about bedtime reading. Careful studies show that the parents read to the children more often and the children end up with larger vocabularies — all for just $20 per child per year. *reachoutandread.org*

SPRINGBOARD COLLABORATIVE provides intensive summer school for disadvantaged children, so that a three-month loss in reading level turns into a 3.3-month gain. A donor can sponsor a child for a summer for $350.

springboardcollaborative.org

SAVE THE CHILDREN provides home visitation, screening and literacy programs for young children. A sponsorship is $28 a month. *savethechildren.org*

Nicholas Kristof, a columnist for The New York Times, and Sheryl WuDunn are the authors of "A Path Appears," from which this essay is adapted.

A version of this op-ed appears in print on September 14, 2014, on page SR1 of the New York edition with the headline: The Way to Beat Poverty.

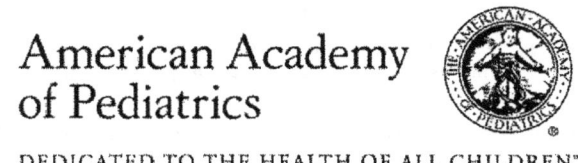

American Academy of Pediatrics

DEDICATED TO THE HEALTH OF ALL CHILDREN™

September 16, 2014

Testimony of
James M. Perrin, MD, FAAP, President

On behalf of the
American Academy of Pediatrics

Before the
Senate Committee on Finance Health Care Subcommittee

American Academy of Pediatrics • Department of Federal Affairs
601 13th Street NW, Suite 400 North • Washington, DC 20005
Tel: 800.336.5475 • E-mail: kids1st@aap.org

My name is Jim Perrin and I join you today on behalf of the 62,000 primary care pediatricians, pediatric subspecialists, and pediatric surgical specialists of the American Academy of Pediatrics. I am a pediatrician from the state of Massachusetts, and am currently the President of the Academy.

Let me begin by thanking you for the opportunity you've afforded the AAP to testify before the Senate Finance Subcommittee on Health Care regarding the Children's Health Insurance Program. Since its bipartisan beginnings, CHIP has developed into a critical program for children and their families. CHIP finances health coverage for over 8 million children across the country and has improved three important aspects of children's health: access to coverage for medical services, utilization of those services, and the population health of millions of children who have benefitted from the program.

Coverage is important for a number of reasons. Uninsured children are three times more likely than children with insurance to lack access to a needed prescription medication, and five times more likely to have an unmet need for medical care. In addition, a just-released CDC report proves that uninsured children receive substantially lower rates of preventive care.

I ask you now to turn your attention to the children you know in your life. As you see with your own eyes, these children are not little adults, and we all know that care for children is different and reflects the realities of children's lives in America. For instance, the number one cause of death in U.S. children is injury, not heart disease or cancer; obesity is epidemic; and children and youth with special health care needs constitute around 15% of the population but 40% of the pediatric "spend."

Children manifest specific characteristics that set them apart from adults. Children depend upon caregivers and other adults to detect medical problems, access health care, translate the nature of their symptoms to clinicians, receive recommendations for care, and arrange for and monitor ongoing treatments.

As infants and children are in constant stages of development, their capabilities, physiology, size, cognitive abilities, judgment, and response to interventions continue to change and require continuous monitoring to ensure that these changes are proceeding within a positive trajectory and that health care is tailored to their developmental stage.

Most children are healthy so that the epidemiology of pediatric disease is different from the adult population. Care for all children is marked by adequate immunization from infectious disease and well baby/well child check-ups to confirm and support healthy development. Nevertheless large and increasing numbers of children have chronic conditions that affect their health and development and require specific care to generate, maintain, and restore age-appropriate functioning to maximize their potential.

Additionally, children are different because they represent the most economically, ethnically, and racially diverse population in the U.S., with very high rates of childhood poverty. Resulting health care disparities put children at risk of adverse outcomes. These specific differences between children and adults require distinct and specific services for infants, children and adolescents that include both preventive care as well as the full range of diagnostic, therapeutic, and ongoing counseling and monitoring of all children, including those with developmental disorders, chronic conditions, behavioral, emotional and learning disabilities.

We have not achieved coverage of these services for every child in the US, but we should all be proud and thankful for the vast strides we have made since SCHIP was established. Today, CHIP is critical in helping to ensure that no child falls through the cracks and that the vast majority of US children have access to the high-quality, affordable health insurance they need and deserve even as poverty in the pediatric population has stubbornly persisted. In fact, even with persistent poverty among children since SCHIP's enactment in 1997, the number of uninsured children has been cut in half, while the number of uninsured adults rose significantly. The reauthorization of the program in 2009 included several improvements, such as improved age-appropriate health benefits, including coverage of dental, mental health, and substance abuse services to the same extent as medical and surgical treatments, and a strong federal investment in child health quality improvement.

The AAP urges Congress to fully fund CHIP through at least 2019, and to do so during this Congress for a host of reasons. Initially, pediatricians are intimately familiar with the interaction between the federal and state governments related to Medicaid and CHIP. States in particular need time to plan and an understanding of what the federal government will do to make wise budgetary decisions. Children and families need the stability that a medical home offers and consistent rules regarding what their insurance covers, the managed care company with whom they will interact and the peace of mind that quality, affordable health care offers. Pediatricians need to know that they will be able to operate their practices with a reliable payer so that they can open their medical home to as many publicly-insured families as possible, recognizing that for too long, private insurance payment rates inadequately offset the low payment rates offered by public payers for so many children. Pediatricians will stretch the dollars that are provided to them, but stability and predictability help any business plan and grow.

CHIP works. For children enrolled in CHIP, most research has found that access to care and utilization of primary and preventive care improve after enrollment. Evaluations conducted in individual states or across combinations of states have found, in general, that enrollees report improvements in having a usual source of care, in completing visits to physicians or dentists, and in having fewer unmet health needs after enrollment. Furthermore, some observers cite evidence indicating that racial/ethnic disparities in access and utilization detectable among new CHIP participants before they enrolled were either eliminated or greatly reduced after enrollment. Other researchers have reported that the benefits of CHIP enrollment with respect to reductions in unmet needs are greater for children with chronic health conditions. Finally, children older than 13 years from low-income families who had not been eligible for public health insurance coverage before the enactment of CHIP appear to have had disproportionately greater increases in the likelihood of a physician visit and greater declines in rates of uninsurance as a result of the enactment of CHIP when compared with younger children from poor and near-poor households.

Finally, over and apart from the direct effects that CHIP has had on the access, utilization, and the health status of near-poor children, the provisions in CHIPRA that focus on the quality of care delivered to children are of signal importance. A major innovative element of CHIPRA was the incorporation of quality child health measurement standards, monitoring capabilities, and reporting requirements for states in Title IV of the Act. CHIPRA established a mechanism by which the Centers for Medicare and Medicaid Services collaborated with the Agency for Healthcare Research and Quality to identify an initial core set of child health quality measures on which states could voluntarily report. CHIPRA also allocated significant catalyzing investments to 10 states – that were collaboratively leveraged by the pediatric community to a total of 18 states – to encourage the creation of on-the-ground quality demonstration projects. In addition, since the law's enactment, the US Department of

Health and Human Services has been required to report on the quality of care received by children covered by Medicaid and CHIP.

CHIP has made important contributions to the advancement of health care delivery to near-poor children in recent years and has the potential to accomplish more in years to come. Going forward, there is a series of issues that the pediatric community must continue to monitor to preserve the advances that have been made and to expand on them where possible. The ACA has mandated that income thresholds for CHIP are to remain constant through 2019 (although Congress has yet to appropriate funds for the program beyond 2015), but state-by-state variability in premiums and cost sharing in the form of deductibles, copayments, and coinsurance for CHIP stand-alone programs will need to be minimized to maintain true access to health care services, especially to subspecialty care.

Congress, the Administration, pediatricians and families must continue to assess vigilantly the comprehensiveness of benefit packages available under the program, because these features will also vary from state to state.

All those with an interest in advancing child well-being should closely monitor eligibility and benefits for emancipated minors, for children up to 26 years of age, for foster children once they reach the age of majority, for children of undocumented immigrants, and other vulnerable populations. Finally, the relationship between CHIP and the new health care marketplaces must be clearly delineated to ensure that the benefits for children are maintained at least at the present level and that the needs of children are not overlooked as these new structures are being created.

The AAP offers the following recommendations to strengthen CHIP for children:
- Fully fund CHIP at least through 2019.
- Expand awareness of CHIP among eligible families.
- Facilitate enrollment in CHIP for eligible children.
- Maximize comprehensive coverage and affordability for children whose care is financed by CHIP dollars.
- Enhance the quality measurement funding established in CHIPRA.
- Ensure adequate payment for physicians who care for CHIP patients.

Children and pediatricians owe tremendous thanks to Senators Rockefeller, Hatch, Wyden, and Roberts for their leadership in working to keep CHIP strong for children. America's pediatricians urge Congress to support the efforts of Senator Rockefeller and others in Congress to continue CHIP's success for at least four more years.

Our country cannot let this program end: families with more than eight million children across the country rely on CHIP to finance their health care coverage, and we owe it to them and our country's future to make sure it continues. Thank you again for all you do for children.

United States Senate Subcommittee on Health
Public Hearing
"The Children's Health Insurance Program: Protecting America's Children and Families"
September 16, 2014

Responses to Questions for the Record From James Perrin

<u>**Senate Finance Committee Chairman Wyden:**</u>

Our health care system is going through a major transition. Americans are gaining access to new coverage options and important protections. As we are navigating this transition, it is imperative that we do not take a step back on children's coverage. As Chairman of the Senate Finance Committee, ensuring kids and their families have access to affordable, comprehensive coverage has and will continue to be a key priority of mine.

Question #1: Dr. Perrin, can you describe the coverage, benefits, and protections children and families receive under the Children's Health Insurance Program and how this compares to other types of health coverage such as qualified health plan or employer sponsored coverage?

Answer: Since it began in 1997, the Children's Health Insurance Program (CHIP) has been a vital health insurance program for children and families, today providing quality health coverage to more than eight million children in families with incomes too high to qualify for Medicaid but too low to afford private health coverage. CHIP typically provides more comprehensive benefits for children than plans available in the Marketplaces. CHIP also protects families' economic security through low out-of-pocket costs. The level of cost sharing and premiums in CHIP vary by state, but families' out-of-pocket expenses cannot exceed 5% of their income. GAO and MACPAC have found that in nearly all instances, CHIP is significantly more affordable than Marketplace coverage. Furthermore, CHIP is designed specifically for children, so its plans include appropriate pediatric providers. In contrast, Marketplace plans often have narrow networks and may not include many pediatric providers.

<u>**Health Subcommittee Chairman Rockefeller:**</u>

During my time as Chair of the Pepper and Children's Commissions, I learned that millions of America's children were falling through the cracks. This reality greatly disturbed me. It seemed unconscionable that millions of children from working families did not have health insurance because they could not afford private coverage—but they were ineligible for Medicaid.
As we now know, the health consequences for children who go without health insurance are significant—and often last in to adulthood. Today, the same families would still be unable to afford health care for their children if it were not for CHIP.

Question #1: Dr. Perrin, in the over 25 years you have been a pediatric health care provider, can you discuss how has the landscape of children's coverage, and quality of that health coverage changed since the bipartisan passage of CHIP?

Answer: Since the bipartisan passage of CHIP in 1997, CHIP, along with Medicaid, has helped to cut the number of low-income, uninsured children across the country by an astonishing 50 percent, while improving health outcomes and access to care. Children now have access to quality health care that was previously unavailable or unaffordable. CHIP enrollees in states that use CHIP funds to grow their Medicaid program are guaranteed the benefits of Medicaid's Early and Periodic Screening, Diagnostic, and Treatment (EPSDT) program, which include health screenings, physical and mental health assessments, laboratory tests including blood lead levels, immunizations, health education; vision, dental, and hearing services; and most importantly, medically necessary treatment for problems found during check-ups.

<u>**Senator Cantwell:**</u>

Question #1: As a pediatrician, can you describe the impact of a disruption of CHIP coverage on a child's health outcomes?

Answer: If CHIP were to be discontinued, many children who are currently enrollees would have to transition to coverage in the Marketplace. Some of these children would have access to subsidies, however others (perhaps more than 2 million children) would fall into what is described as a "family glitch." In other words, they would not be eligible for subsidized coverage through the Marketplace if they have access to employer-sponsored coverage through a parent, even if that coverage is unaffordable. This would leave them without health insurance and would certainly contribute to poorer health outcomes. It would also likely disrupt their access to the medical home they may have had for quite some time. In pediatrics, a medical home is not a building, house, hospital, or home healthcare service, but rather an approach to providing comprehensive primary care. In a medical home, the pediatric care team works in partnership with a child and a child's family to assure that all of the medical and non-medical needs of the patient are met. Through this partnership the pediatric care team can help the family/patient access, coordinate, and understand specialty care, educational services, out-of-home care, family support, and other public and private community services that are important for the overall health of the child and family. The American Academy of Pediatrics (AAP) developed the medical home model for delivering primary care that is accessible, continuous, comprehensive, family-centered, coordinated, compassionate, and culturally effective to all children and youth, including children and youth with special health care needs. Disrupting a child's medical home by ending CHIP could be problematic for their continuity of care. Furthermore, children transitioning from CHIP to QHPs would likely experience a reduction in covered child-specific benefits and increased cost sharing, which could also worsen their health outcomes.

Opening Statement
Senate Finance Subcommittee Hearing
The Children's Health Insurance Program: Protecting America's Children and Families
Senator John D. Rockefeller IV
September 16, 2014

I have proudly served on the Finance committee for almost every one of my thirty years in the Senate and I have chaired or been ranking member of this subcommittee for twenty of those years.

This will be the last Health Subcommittee hearing I chair, and I could not think of a more important subject to discuss today than children's health care.

2014 marks the 17th anniversary of one of the most successful programs for improving children's health in the United States: the Children's Health Insurance Program—more commonly referred to as "CHIP."

Eight million American children and families look to CHIP for comprehensive and affordable health coverage, including 40,000 children in my home state of West Virginia. CHIP's success has played an essential role in cutting the number of uninsured children in half over the past 15 years.

This kind of progress is something we should celebrate. But, we must continue to invest in CHIP so that we can celebrate many more of the program's milestones.

In 1997, Senators Kennedy and Hatch and I spent countless hours discussing how we could increase health care access for children in a way that members of both political parties could support. CHIP was the result of those conversations.

Creating this program has been one of the most impactful things I have done in my career in public service. Safeguarding CHIP so that it can live on for years to come is my highest priority in the time I have left in office.

Without Congressional action, CHIP will run out of funding next fall, placing at risk the well-being of hundreds of thousands of children and pregnant women. I hope that the members of this committee will not let that happen.

CHIP is a game-changer for millions of children. No other form of coverage provides the same level of specific care and comprehensive pediatric networks at an affordable cost for working families.

The challenges many children face today are still too similar to the ones I saw firsthand in Emmons, West Virginia 50 years ago. It was there in southern West Virginia where I witnessed the struggles that families go through when they can't afford health care for their children.

When I first arrived as a VISTA volunteer in Emmons, there were children in the town and across the state who had never seen a doctor because their families simply didn't have the money to cover the costs of a physician visit or dental care.

I thought to myself then, as I still do now, that no parent should have to carry the stress of knowing you cannot afford health care for your child if something goes wrong.

I'm proud to say that ever since CHIP's inception, the program has consistently enjoyed strong bipartisan support. One member of the Finance Committee—Senator Hatch—has remained a steadfast champion for CHIP from the beginning.

We have a shared goal of making certain that every child in America gets a fair shot at a healthy start in life. While we have not always agreed on every provision in the CHIP program, I have always appreciated Senator Hatch's strong commitment to CHIP.

For as long as I can recall, Congress has been able to put aside its differences and come together when it's called upon to do what's right for America's children. And that time has come again.

CHIP is currently at a crossroads. Funding for CHIP must be reauthorized soon; otherwise, the program as we know it will come to an end. As many as two million children could lose their insurance coverage.

This would threaten their health and well-being, not to mention the significant gains we've made over the past 17 years to reduce the number of uninsured children and youth in this country. We simply cannot afford to take this major step backwards and jeopardize our future generations by allowing CHIP to expire.

A recent study by Wakely Consulting Group demonstrated that moving children into other forms of private coverage could cause a ten-fold increase of out-of-pocket spending for CHIP families.

It is not right to shift added financial burden onto working families when a cost-effective solution for maintaining the coverage they already have for their children exists.

Although funding for CHIP expires in 2015, the program is authorized through 2019. Ending the program prior to 2019 could therefore lead to significant disruption for state governments, private health plans, hospitals, and numerous other stakeholders in addition to the families whose children are enrolled in the program. States have been budgeting and planning under the assumption that Congress will extend funding for another four years.

They simply are not prepared to rapidly develop and implement plans to transition millions of children into other forms of coverage. In short, state legislatures and budget offices are relying on us to act now.

Colleagues, let's do our job today. Let's show the American people that we are committed to the health and well-being of our youngest generation and extend the Children's Health Insurance Program.

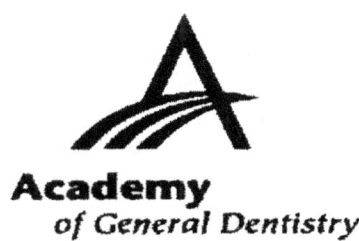

Academy
of General Dentistry

September 16, 2014

The Honorable Jay Rockefeller
Chairman
Senate Finance Subcommittee on Health Care
United States Senate
Washington, DC 20510

**Re: Subcommittee Hearing: The Children's Health Insurance Program:
Protecting America's Children and Families**

Dear Senator Rockefeller:

On behalf of the Academy of General Dentistry's (AGD) 38,000 membership
network, I am pleased to offer the following comments for the record with regard to
the September 16 hearing of the Subcommittee entitled, "The Children's Health
Insurance Program: Protecting America's Children and Families."

The AGD commends you for taking action to improve the oral health of our nation's
children with your legislation, S. 2461, the CHIP Extension Act of 2014. Failure to
extend the Children's Health Insurance Program (CHIP) would be devastating to the
millions of at-risk children in need of affordable oral health services. It is important
to note, however, that while access to affordable treatment represents an important
piece of the oral health care equation, a renewed emphasis on oral health literacy is
urgently needed to fully address the problem of chronic oral health ailments in our
country.

As you know, the Children's Health Insurance Program Reauthorization Act of 2009
(CHIPRA) guaranteed CHIP enrolled children access to comprehensive and
affordable dental coverage. This coverage has enabled families to obtain the care
needed to prevent and treat dental disease. Under CHIP, annual costs are based on
income, making it easier for families to afford coverage. The AGD especially
appreciates the explicit recognition that inclusion of dental care in the five percent
cost-sharing limit is critical to the affordability of health coverage for working
families.

As mentioned, the AGD feels strongly that the importance of prevention in the form
of oral health literacy is often overlooked, much to the detriment of our nation's oral
health needs. Studies have shown that the public is largely unaware of the

connection between oral health and overall health and well being. Yet the fact remains that a vast majority of oral health ailments can be avoided by increasing oral health literacy among all populations, with a special emphasis on children to ensure they develop and maintain healthy habits into adulthood. Recognizing that many oral disease ailments are preventable, we feel that more needs to be done at all levels to educate the public about the importance of maintaining good oral health.

Like you, the AGD shares a strong commitment to improving essential health and oral health care for all individuals, especially those in high-risk populations. To that end, the AGD stands ready to work with you and your staff to generate support for S. 2461. Further, we look forward to serving as a resource for you on future initiatives aimed at improving oral health and oral health access. Please do not hesitate to contact Daniel J. Buksa, JD, Associate Executive Director, Public Affairs, by phone at 312.440.4328 or via email at Daniel.buksa@agd.org to let us know how we may be of further assistance.

Thank you again for your efforts regarding this critical issue.

Sincerely,

W. Carter Brown, DMD, FAGD
President
Academy of General Dentistry

cc: Members of the Senate Finance Subcommittee on Health Care

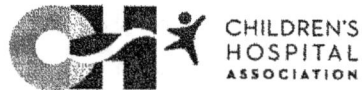

CHILDREN'S HOSPITAL ASSOCIATION

For Immediate Release
September 16, 2014

Contact: Tim Haynes
timothy.haynes@childrenshospitals.org
202-753-5372

Children's Hospitals Applaud Senators for Highlighting Importance of CHIP
Senate Finance Subcommittee on Health Care Hearing Looks at Protecting America's Children

WASHINGTON, DC — The Children's Hospital Association thanks Sens. John D. Rockefeller IV (D-WV) and Pat Roberts (R-KS) for holding a hearing on the important and unique role the Children's Health Insurance Program (CHIP) plays in protecting America's children and families.

Health care providers, like state budget offices and millions of families around the country, are looking to Congress to provide certainty about the future of the program before year's end. Unless Congress intervenes, CHIP's funding will expire in September 2015, disrupting coverage for a projected 10 million children. If CHIP expires, the impact on state budgets could exceed a combined loss of $1 billion annually, effectively shifting costs to states. As a result, states could be forced to pass these costs onto providers and families or further shift costs in ways that jeopardize low-income children's access to care.

Children's hospitals support a timely extension of CHIP through FY2019 and applaud bipartisan lawmakers in both the House and Senate who have worked in recent months to actively engage on the future of CHIP. The Association urges all members of Congress to work towards enactment of legislation extending CHIP to ensure continued availability of stable coverage to meet the unique needs of children.

Since its bipartisan beginning in 1997, CHIP has maintained a proven track record providing pediatric-specific care including developmentally-appropriate benefits, a full range of providers in network and affordable cost-sharing protections. Further, it has spurred highly successful state outreach and enrollment strategies to get eligible children enrolled in Medicaid and CHIP coverage. As a result, children's uninsurance has dropped to the lowest level on record in history.

The Association also highlights the importance of continuing the first significant national investment in pediatric quality, enacted under the CHIP Reauthorization Act of 2009, to close the gap in quality measurement and improvement between children and adults. This pediatric quality funding has spurred the creation and stewardship of maternal and child health quality measures in addition to 10 demonstration projects that are working to lower costs and improve outcomes for maternal and child health populations across 18 states. Extending this funding in tandem with a CHIP extension would foster continued progress towards obtaining effective measures of child health quality that can be used across multiple payers to improve child health outcomes.

###

Children's Hospital Association advances child health through innovation in the quality, cost and delivery of care. Representing more than 220 children's hospitals, the Association is the voice of children's hospitals nationally. The Association champions public policies that enable hospitals to better serve children, and is the premier resource for pediatric data and analytics driving clinical and operational performance of members hospitals. www.childrenshospitals.org | www.speaknowforkids.org

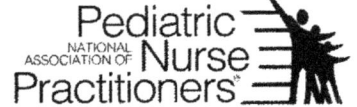

Headquarters
5 Hanover Square
Suite 1401
New York, NY 10004
P.917-746-8300
www.napnap.org

Government Affairs Office
20 F St. NW
Suite 700
Washington, D.C. 20001
P. 202-223-2250

"The Children's Health Insurance Program: Protecting America's Children and Families"

The United States Senate Committee on Finance

Subcommittee on Health Care

September 16, 2014

Submitted for the Hearing Record by the

National Association of Pediatric Nurse Practitioners

Mary L. Chesney, PhD, RN, CPNP, President

Chairman Rockefeller, Senator Roberts and distinguished members of the Subcommittee:

On behalf of 7,800 pediatric nurse practitioners (PNPs) committed to providing optimal health care to children, the National Association of Pediatric Nurse Practitioners (NAPNAP) thanks you for holding this important and timely hearing on the future of the Children's Health Insurance Program. We join our colleagues and children's health advocates everywhere in recognizing Senator Rockefeller for his years of tireless service and commitment to improving the health of all Americans – particularly the millions of children who have been the beneficiaries of his leadership in creating the CHIP program.

Pediatric nurse practitioners are licensed advanced practice nurses who have enhanced education in pediatric health care and extensive practice and policy experience with both the Medicaid and Children's Health Insurance Program (CHIP). PNPs have been providing quality primary care, specialty, and acute care to children and families for more than 40 years in an extensive range of practice settings such as pediatric offices, schools and hospitals – reaching millions of patients across the country each year. PNPs provide care to newborns, infants, children, adolescents and young adults that includes health and developmental screening, managing acute and chronic conditions, ordering and interpreting diagnostic tests, prescribing medications, administering immunizations, coordinating care across the health care continuum and making referrals to other professionals as appropriate.

PNPs know first-hand how important the CHIP program is to the health of children in our country. CHIP has become a dependable source of coverage for low-income children in working families whose parents earn too much to qualify for Medicaid but too little to afford private health insurance. Since 1997 when CHIP was enacted with strong bipartisan support, it has helped to cut the number of low-income, uninsured children across the country by an amazing 50 percent – from 25 percent in 1997 to 13 percent in 2012 – while improving health outcomes and access to care for children and pregnant women. More than 8 million children across the country were insured through CHIP in 2012 – an all-time high.

The services that CHIP helps to provide are crucial for children's health. Uninsured children are three times more likely that those with insurance to lack needed medication and five times more likely to have an unmet health care need, including significantly lower rates of preventive care. Children enrolled in CHIP have access to a full range of primary, specialty and ancillary pediatric providers, including pediatric nurse practitioners, to ensure they receive comprehensive medically and developmentally appropriate care.

The CHIP program helps to ensure that low-income families have access to affordable care by limiting their out-of-pocket costs to no more than 5 percent of family income. In addition, many states provide children enrolled in CHIP with Medicaid's Early and Periodic Screening, Diagnostic and Treatment (EPSDT) benefit, a strong set of pediatric-specific benefits that provides comprehensive care based on children's unique needs.

As you know, one of the strengths of the CHIP program is a structure that gives states flexibility to design a program that meets the needs of their distinct populations. This design has helped states tackle the costs of uncompensated care while reducing the numbers of uninsured children and pregnant women. The number of children eligible for but not enrolled children in Medicaid and CHIP dropped by 18 percent between 2008 and 2011 – thanks largely to flexible state options created by Congress to improve enrollment strategies, such as express lane eligibility and 12-month continuous eligibility, when the CHIP program was last reauthorized in 2009. At the same time, because CHIP is a program devised specifically for children, its benefit design and provider networks are tailored to meet their special needs.

NAPNAP believes that continued federal funding for CHIP is essential to maintain these gains in health care coverage for children. As you are well aware, although Congress has authorized the program itself through federal fiscal year 2019, federal funding for the program will expire on October 1, 2015 unless Congress takes action to extend it. At a time when states are still adjusting to numerous changes in health care coverage, PNPs believe it is essential that Congress secure CHIP's future this year, so that states will be able to operate their programs without disruption. Without CHIP, the uninsured rate would increase significantly and the health of children and families would be jeopardized. The Congressional Budget Office recently estimated that 12.7 million children projected to be enrolled in fiscal year 2015 are at risk of losing their CHIP coverage in 2016 if the program is not reauthorized. Likewise, pregnant women enrolled in CHIP could be left without other sources of prenatal care, jeopardizing the health of their newborns.

CHIP typically provides more comprehensive benefits designed to meet children's needs than plans offered in health insurance marketplaces. At least half of the states have chosen as their benchmark the "largest small business plan" primarily designed for adults. In nearly all instances, CHIP is substantially more affordable than current marketplace policies and provides better coverage for children. Finally, the so-called "family glitch" means that families that include as many as 2 million children who would otherwise be eligible will not be able to obtain premium tax credits to purchase affordable marketplace health coverage.

NAPNAP is grateful to Chairman Rockefeller for introducing the "CHIP Extension Act" (S. 2461) and for convening this hearing to begin this critically important discussion on a bipartisan approach to preserving and improving children's health care by continuing the Children's Health Insurance Program. Pediatric nurse practitioners look forward to working with you and your colleagues to take prompt action to extend the CHIP program before the end of this year.